MW01282708

I Can See The Moon, But Not The Stars

A Memoir by
CARMELA CANTISANI

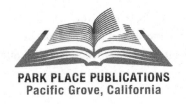

PARK PLACE PUBLICATIONS
Pacific Grove, California

DEDICATION

This book is dedicated to the apple of my eye, my husband, best friend, and the love of my life, Gilbert Converset. Shortly after we met, he undertook the enormous challenge over the course of two years not only to learn how to ski–my favorite obsession—but to become my skiing guide.

From our wedding in a hot air balloon, to our many travels and adventures over lands and seas, multiple professional assignments, difficult family dynamics and deaths, he has given me his vision of the world in a more profound way than most husbands could ever do. His patience and kind response to my tumultuous character and occasional frustrations have allowed me to achieve the peaceful stability I had been so yearning for.

Gilbert, I am so grateful to you for giving me the opportunity to publish this autobiography and for the vision we share!

I Can See The Moon, But Not The Stars
A Memoir by Carmela Cantisani

Second Edition August 02 , 2023 (Edited by Terry Nelson)
© 2022 Carmela Cantisani
ISBN 13: 978-1-953120-40-3
Interior Design and Format
Patricia Hamilton
Published by
Park Place Publications
Pacific Grove, California
www.parkplacepublications.com
Photographs from the Cantisani Family Collection.

CONTENTS

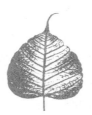

ACKNOWLEDGEMENTS AND DISCLAIMER

This book could not have happened without the assistance and enthusiastic encouragement of a great many people, only a few of whom I can mention here.

I wrote the first few paragraphs of this book on an airplane with my Braille hand slate on 3x5 cards. After that initial start, it became a team effort with my husband, Gilbert, who entered my words from Braille to an e-version. With his help, my thoughts turned into coherent paragraphs, and a rough draft began to take shape.

Gilbert's technical assistance and continual support was invaluable during this project; and words cannot express my deeply felt appreciation.

I have profound gratitude to Signe Thorsen, a treasured friend, who was instrumental in bringing this book to life. Her keen eye and sense of language were evident when she typed my first dictation. "You've started your book, now you just have to finish it," Signe said. Since those initial days her support has been unflagging. She is a seeker of truth and clarity who pushed, cajoled, and encouraged me to get my story right. To Signe, who was always wise, and always available, I will be forever grateful.

Very special thanks to my life-long family friend and accomplished writer, Lee Marcus, who read my material at its roughest stage and gave me the firm but supportive push I needed to move this book forward. Lee helped me bring to completion my first coherent draft during a memorable transatlantic cruise from Fort Lauderdale to Rome, and for that I am deeply appreciative.

Long-time friends, Donna Bickelmann, Debra Thomas, and Vivian Picow, provided valuable support when my confidence needed a boost. My gratitude to all of them. Thanks, also, to Maryellen Eisenberg,

Sylvie Reynolds, and Beverly Klayman for helping with the book's final touches.

With heartfelt love and sincere gratitude, I thank my family, both immediate and extended, for providing support and details about generations that I have never known. What happened to them before my birth shaped who I am today and gave me the inspiration for this book.

To those individuals mentioned, and those who are not … you are far from forgotten. *I Can See The Moon, But Not The Stars* came to be because of you. We are partners in this writing endeavor, and I am honored to take this opportunity to acknowledge you.

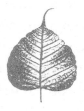

PROLOGUE

On January 1st 1999, I flew home to Monterey, California, after a usual holiday visit with my family in Westchester County, New York. I had been taking frequent trips to New York in recent years to spend more time with my aging, ailing parents. My two older siblings, Benny and Maria, who still lived in Westchester County, were responsible for providing my parents' day-to-day support.

My immediate family had emigrated from Southern Italy to the Westchester area in the mid-1960s. We were following in the footsteps of members of my mother's extended family who had emigrated over the past several decades from the same region. I left Westchester in 1972 to attend the Monterey Institute of International Studies in Monterey, California. After I graduated with a degree in French, the Monterey Peninsula became my permanent home.

Just a few days after I returned from my trip, I received word that my 85-year-old father had died. Seven years prior, my father had suffered a debilitating stroke which left him paralyzed on the left side of his body. I was devastated. If only I had remained in New York just a little longer, I would have been there when he was hospitalized and I could have been with him until the end.

As I made my way back east to attend his funeral, I was on the same flight as my younger brother Peter, my only sibling living in California, and my husband, Gilbert Converset. I felt comforted being with them during this difficult time.

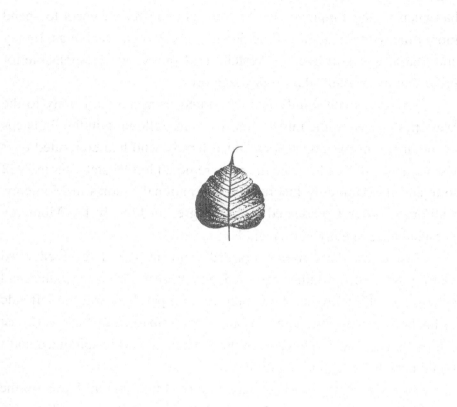

CHAPTER 1

MY FATHER'S FUNERAL

My father's funeral was held on a perfect winter day. The air was still, snow fell steadily, the trees stood tall and proud, elegantly dressed in white suits. New Yorkers had succumbed to the will of nature. They drove slowly and moved about gingerly as if everything were a well-rehearsed opening scene to my father's funeral procession.

As the driver carefully inched forward behind the hearse, I sat quietly in the limousine listening to the soothing chatter of the snowflakes on the window. I thought of my early childhood years—the only time I really got to spend with my family. Those years I lived so close to my mother and father are precious to me because at the age of five I was sent away to boarding school and never lived at home full-time again.

During my early childhood, home was a two-room farmhouse secluded in the high hills of the Basilicata region of Southern Italy. The conditions were simple, even primitive. We slept on corn husk mattresses, had no running water, no electricity, and no paved roads for miles. I thought the whole world was like that and I was happy.

On cold, snowy mornings, my father would be the first one up. He would carve his way to the nearby shed and pick up some dry wood for a fire. My older brother Biagio slept in the hayloft above the livestock barn since there was no room for him in the house. He joined my father in gathering firewood.

As soon as the fire crackled to life, my mother would start cooking breakfast, which would take at least an hour to prepare. The younger siblings, not yet old enough to be useful, waited in bed. Not only was it the warmest spot in the house, but staying out of the way of adults who were hectically working on important tasks was the smart thing to do.

My mother would boil water in a heavy kettle on a tripod over the fire and make polenta with our homegrown corn flour. We ate polenta nearly every day. The only thing that changed was the seasoning and topping, and it was always delicious.

My parents' main occupation was the care and nurturing of their family, and how lucky we were for that. Now, half a century later, on this snowy ride to Ferncliff Cemetery, the wonderfully warm and vital man who had been my father belonged to me only in sweet memory, which made me weep.

During the wake at the funeral home the day before, a steady stream of family members, friends, neighbors, co-workers, and acquaintances young and old had come by to pay their last respects to my father. Of course, the immediate family was out in full force: my mother Rosa, eighty-one years old, all my siblings with their respective families, my husband, Gilbert Converset, and me.

An impressive number of mourners came to the wake. My intellectual side unfortunately wouldn't shut off and it made me feel somewhat uncomfortable. I couldn't help noticing the unintentional hypocrisy of this tradition. If all of these people who came to see my father now had taken the time to visit him in the nursing home during the last three years of his life, he would have had a visitor nearly every day.

Of course the idea of visiting patients in any kind of hospital may have still been foreign to many of my father's contemporaries. There were no nursing homes for the elders in Italy. They died most often in their own beds, surrounded by family and friends. The priest would have come and administered Last Rites, and all would have been familiar and in order.

At the funeral home before they closed the casket, I wiped away my tears with a small, embroidered handkerchief I'd had since I was a child. I placed the handkerchief in the left pocket of his shirt under his jacket, and said goodbye to my father.

During the church service following the wake, I found little comfort in the words recited by the Catholic priest. I wanted at all costs to believe that someday I would see my father again and that God would take good care of his soul until then.

If only I could have stopped analyzing everything I was hearing in the priest's sermon, perhaps I could have felt somewhat at peace like everyone else seemed to be. But, if I did see my father again in the afterlife, what would he be like? Would he be young or old? Would he be my father without his faults? Would he no longer take God's name in vain, or swear at my mother for being a backseat driver? Would I recognize my father if he behaved like a well-mannered "Heavenite"?

After we laid my father to rest in the Ferncliff Cemetery, family and friends gathered at a local Italian-American restaurant for a meal. With a heavy heart I pondered unanswerable questions. Who are we? Where do we come from and why are we here? What is life, really, and what is death?

Within a day or two after my father's funeral, everyone who had come from out-of-town went back home to resume their lives. I chose to remain in New York. I needed to get used to the new family structure with my father absent.

Early the next morning while I was still in bed, I heard my mother in the kitchen, weeping. I quietly entered the room and sat next to her at the table, gently stroking her thick, well-coiffed hair. She held her head between her hands and muttered, "If only my father had not returned us to Italy when I was a child, so much pain and suffering could have been avoided." I knew exactly what she meant. Her life had not turned out to be at all what she had hoped.

CHAPTER 2

MY MOTHER

Rosa Cantisani had given birth to six children. The first two of whom were sighted and the last four were blind, one of whom died at birth. I happened to be one of the blind children. We blind kids certainly bore some of the burden for her misfortune. Both of my parents, to different degrees, were unable to move past our "disability," no matter what we did.

The bottom line for them was that however clever, talented, or successful we became, even as professionals, we would still have been better off sighted. They failed to see the benefits that came with our blindness. It was due to our blindness that they had the opportunity to learn new things, explore new parts of the world, good and bad, and expand their horizons in so many ways.

For years, this subject of blindness was taboo in my presence. Because I would become so adamant about my point of view, the discussion would always deteriorate into a huge argument resulting in a long period of tension between us.

This time, though, I allowed my mother to grieve in peace. She went through her litany of reasons why her life had been miserable, and how much better off she would have been had she had the chance to grow up in America instead of returning to Italy as a young child. For one, her education would have gone past grade school and she would not have felt like a second-class citizen due to her lack of education. Two, she certainly would have married a different man, not given birth to blind children, and therefore all the circumstances surrounding her married life would have been different. Different, certainly. Better? Not necessarily, I thought.

For the previous two years or so, my mother had been gradually exhibiting changes in personality. Unlike the rest of the family, I was not attributing these changes to my father's long illness or just to old age, but to Alzheimer's disease (which would be confirmed about a year later). Because I held this suspicion, I didn't become impatient when she repeated questions or told the same stories over and over.

From research, I learned how the Alzheimer's disease progresses, so I wanted to make sure her stories were told before it would be too late. I knew how to fill in the gaps when her memories failed her and as a result she seemed more at ease talking to me now than she had ever been in the past. It was important to me to spend time with her every single day so that I could really find out about her life beyond what I already knew. I quickly realized that she enjoyed it very much and it seemed to be therapeutic for both of us.

While I was in New York, another of my goals was to discuss with my sister Maria the possibility of locating a good daycare center for our mother. She needed a place where she could spend time participating in stimulating activities so she wouldn't remain idle and wither away watching mindless TV programs. My mother always liked to be active and spend her time socializing, but with my father's long illness, she had grown tired and depressed. This was exacerbated when we had to put my father into a nursing home four years into his illness.

"Is this a dignified way to die? If I get to the point where I can no longer take good care of myself," she would say, "please throw me into a ditch and let me die in peace; but no daycare center and no nursing home for me!"

For years, my blind brothers and I had tried in vain to convince our parents to purchase long-term health insurance. "I'm not going to believe in a million years that in America, they would abandon old people when they get sick," my father would say, dismissing all of our arguments. "We have Medicare, plus the supplemental insurance from the union. That's more than enough," he would continue confidently.

My parents had never imagined that one day one of them would get sick, and in order to receive coverage and assistance, they would first have to use up all of their savings and assets—all of the money they worked so hard to save their entire life.

My brother Peter, who has a lot more patience than I do, would use scenarios to explain how the health care system works in America. "Medicare pays only up to a point. If you get sick with a long-term condition, you have to use up all of your savings first before you can receive any assistance from the government. Trust me, that's how it works."

"First of all, it doesn't make any sense to me, but even if it does work like that, what makes you think we would get sick? If we do get sick, we'll deal with it then," said my father.

"You just have to pray to God we don't get sick," said my mother.

"God is not going to come down and pay your hospital bills, trust me," said Peter.

Whether they prayed to God or not, it did happen to them and they were devastated both emotionally and financially. Their American dreams came crashing down when my father suffered a massive stroke seven years prior to his death.

It sickened me to realize that the progression of her disease was forcing us to go against her wishes on this matter. I was convinced, however, that with the right type of stimulation and company, she would start to come around. After reviewing several recommended activity centers geared to the elderly in an early stage of Alzheimer's, Maria and I settled on one of them and arranged to spend a day there with her to see how she would do.

Once we were at the center, she seemed to be herself. She said hello to people and was sociable. We had lunch, which she liked. This was already a big hurdle because she was usually critical of food that was not homemade. After lunch, the staff gathered the patients in the recreation room and put on some upbeat Latin music. At that point, my mother started smiling, stood up and made small steps to the beat of the music. One of the staff invited her to the dance floor and she was delighted. My mother was always happiest when she was surrounded by people, and truly happy if dancing was involved. I felt uplifted seeing her having so much fun. For sure this is the right place for her. She could have the time of her life here, I thought. Pretty soon a lot of the other guests and staffers joined in.

Maria and I decided to step away and observe our mother from a distance to see how she did without us in her view. Based on what we were seeing, it seemed like we had found the right place. There were other Italian guests with whom she could converse, and she was having fun.

But before long, her demeanor changed. She seemed confused and lost among people she didn't recognize. She looked around bewildered, probably asking herself, "What am I doing here? Who are these people? How did I get here?"

The staff tried to redirect her attention, but she pulled away and started running around as if she were looking for someone she recognized. She became more and more agitated and started screaming, "Where is my family? Where are my daughters? Where are my children? What am I doing here? This is not my house!"

Maria and I could no longer watch without intervening. As my mother's primary caregiver, Maria was used to coming to the rescue. As for me, there was something all too familiar and painful about this scene. It stirred memories of the first day I was separated from my parents and forced to enter boarding school at age five. My panic and rage at that time was almost exactly what I was witnessing now. We quickly approached my mother and calmed her down. We took her home and decided to postpone daycare for the time being.

I would be spending the next several weeks with my mother in New York. I had plenty of time to scrutinize her disease and better assess her needs for when we decided to try this again. Within a day or two, my sister and her husband left for a week in Florida. My sister's two grown children, Rosie and Frank, who still lived at home, would join us for dinner every evening, but otherwise my mother and I would be spending all day together with only each other for company.

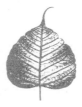

CHAPTER 3

STROLLING WITH SECRETS

The day after Maria and Tony left for Florida, I thought it would be the perfect time to go on a short stroll with my mother around my sister's property. After our morning *café latte*, I told my mother to get bundled up for a walk. She was always eager to be outdoors on a nice day.

"Wow. It's sunny, but the air is really cold. Brrr!" she said, snuggling into her winter scarf.

I grabbed her elbow and away we went. As we were walking along the driveway, she commented on the neat piles of snow that her grandson, Frank, had made with the snowplow. She began fiddling with her coat buttons and scanning around with her eyes as though she were looking for something in particular. After a bit, she said, "During the spring, that whole side of the property gets filled with beautiful flowers."

My mother loved flowers. And so, to encourage the conversation, I said, "Which side of the property are you referring to? This side or that side?"

"Right there, where I am pointing," she said. "Why are you looking the other way?"

My blood went cold. Oh no, I thought, don't tell me she is forgetting I am blind. This was a disaster. I had left the house as an irresponsible blind person. I had not bothered to take my white cane, my guide dog, or my cell phone. I had ignored an important lesson many of my teachers had tried to drill into me for years and years: never relinquish your safety and independence to others. Period!

I had not really given it a second thought; it was my mother I was walking with, after all. I had never worried in the past that I would be in danger while in the company of my own mother. I knew my way around the property, but what if I tripped on something because my mother was no longer automatically looking out for me?

As we moved closer to the street, the more fidgety my mother became. She would take a few steps forward, then stop and look around as though she didn't quite recognize her surroundings.

"What's the matter?" I asked.

"Where did we end up?" she questioned. "Why are we here?"

I tried to reassure her of her whereabouts, but to no avail. Her body was tense, her hands clutched together, her stare fixed on something across the street. She looked across the way and exclaimed, "My children! My children! They're in that building over there. I have to go and get them."

"Which children? Your grandchildren?" I asked, almost in a panic.

"No!" she responded, "My children! They put my children in that building. I have to get to them."

Now I was really panicking. My mother, for the first time in my experience, was exhibiting a full memory lapse and I had no idea how to deal with the situation. I realized I was hearing, perhaps for the first time, my mother's side of a painful story we shared. Something she saw in that house across from my sister's must have reminded her of the school my blind brothers and I had attended so long ago in Naples, Italy. Back then, my mother had to choose as the lesser of two evils to send her three youngest children off to a residential school for the blind where they could get an education.

It was apparent that this experience must have been more traumatic to her than I had known. Up until then, I had always assumed that my pain at being separated from my family had been greater than hers. In her present confusion she was becoming so agitated that I was afraid she would run across the street.

Somehow, I managed to change the subject by saying, "Mom, let's go back inside. Aunt Mary's coming to visit. Remember? We have to get some coffee and cookies ready." My mother loved company, so this ploy worked; it got her attention and we got back inside safely. I locked all the doors, and from then on I kept a very keen ear to her whereabouts.

For the rest of that day I struggled to grasp what had happened that morning. Obviously, my mother's disease was more advanced than I had realized. I didn't know how prolonged or permanent this memory loss was or how much it encompassed. But in her confusion, bits and pieces of painful memories were surfacing, giving me unexpected access to her once-guarded feelings. It soon dawned on me that there might be a positive side to all of this. If she was beginning to forget that three of her children were blind, then possibly her decades of guilt and so much grief were also coming to an end.

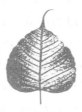

CHAPTER 4

MEET MY MATERNAL GRANDPARENTS

My maternal grandparents, Petronilla and Pietro Cosentino, married in 1900, in the Basilicata region of Southern Italy, where they had been born. Their first child, Giacinta (later Jenny, in English), was born in 1901. Soon after her birth, my grandfather set out for his first trip to New York, along with other men from the area who were able to emigrate. Some of these men were our close relatives.

During those years a virtual wave of men left the poorer regions of Southern Italy to immigrate to the United States. For some, they considered this a permanent move. For others like my grandfather, they left their homeland to find work, earn as much money as they could, then return to their families and provide a better life for them.

My grandfather returned to Italy a couple of years later and stayed long enough to father two more children, Feluccia and Maria. By about 1910, my grandparents decided that he would return to New York one more time. On this trip he tried to convince my grandmother to join him, but he was not successful. My grandmother was not keen on the idea of going to America, coping with a new world and all of its uncertainties. The world as she knew it was good enough for her.

Petronilla lived surrounded by her family and she had the emotional support she needed. The entire farm community was integrated in all aspects of everyone's lives, working together to make life easier for each individual. They helped each other raise the children, manage the farms, plant and harvest the crops, feed and take care of the livestock. The work was hard, but together they made it happen. It would have been a colossal sacrifice for any mother to give that up. Petronilla hoped my grandfather would reconsider the decision to bring the family to America. She hoped he would follow his fatherly instincts, make the money he wanted to make, start missing his family, and come back home. Unfortunately, this did not happen.

In America, my grandfather and many other Italian immigrants were hired on a construction crew to build the Mount Carmel Church on Park Hill Avenue in Yonkers, New York. He was part of the crew that laid the first bricks for the foundation of the building. As my grandfather kept busy working on the church, my grandmother was back in Italy, very busy raising three girls.

Time passed and World War I threatened. Soon enough it became obvious my grandmother was not winning the argument with my grandfather. He didn't seem to be making plans to return to Italy as she had hoped. One day she received a letter from her brother, who was also living in New York and working on the church alongside my grandfather.

He wrote, "You better make plans to join your husband in New York soon, or you might lose him to a woman who has been buzzing around him for quite some time." That was all my grandmother needed to hear. Suddenly she was motivated to join her husband and began making preparations necessary for herself and her three children to make the long journey to the New World.

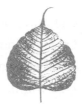

CHAPTER 5

LEAVING BEHIND, MOVING FORWARD

As the departure date neared in February of 1915, Petronilla found herself going about her chores with tears in her eyes. Her heart was filled with melancholy. In those days, when emigrating families said goodbye to their loved ones it was for good. They had no expectation of seeing each other again. She would be leaving behind the only world she had ever known. Nevertheless, filled with faith and hope for a better tomorrow for her children, she kept moving forward. The children, of course, were excited as children always are when about to embark on a new adventure.

In preparation for the journey, they got up before dawn and loaded up the mules and donkeys with their luggage and children. The two youngest rode in baskets that hung on either side of the saddle. My grandmother, her parents, her siblings, and any friends who could be away from home for the day walked from the farm to the town of Castelluccio Inferiore, where everything was unloaded from the animals and transferred to a bus. At the bus stop she had to say goodbye to a good number of her entourage who were unable to accompany her any further.

The bus took her and the children to the train station, at least an hour away from Castelluccio. Once on the train only a couple of family members were able to continue the trip with her all the way to the port of Naples where they wished Petronilla and her daughters a tearful farewell.

The family boarded a ship in Naples for the long, hard voyage. Once on board, a bunk bed was waiting for them in steerage where they would sleep for the next month. All emigrants traveled in steerage in those days. The men were segregated into one dorm, women and children in another. The conditions were unsanitary, overcrowded, and foul-smelling. The meals were miserly and the travelers were not treated well by the staff. Everyone was anxious and apprehensive. In addition, the weather was stormy and they were all seasick for many days.

In spite of the anxiousness and apprehension that I am sure dominated the thoughts of every passenger in steerage, they became supportive of each other as the days passed. As they got to know one another, their local dialects immediately identified where each family originated. They shared family stories as they tried to fill the long, monotonous, and unpleasant days.

I imagine that my grandmother spent countless hours wondering what really lay ahead in her future and praying that they would all arrive in New York safely. She was heartsick about everything she had left behind as all emigrants are.

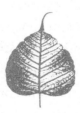

CHAPTER 6

ADJUSTING TO A NEW LIFE

Once in America the Cosentino family of five settled into a modest apartment on Oak Street in Yonkers. Adjusting to their new life in New York and living with the man of the house (my grandfather) for the first time in so long was challenging for my grandmother. But being in a community of mostly immigrants from poor areas of Southern Italy gave them a comforting sense of belonging, which is priceless in a strange land.

The younger girls—Maria, eight and Feluccia, six—were enrolled in school. The older daughter, Giacinta, at fourteen was too old to attend school, but not old enough to work. However, she needed to do something to contribute to the family earnings. My crafty grandfather fiddled around with her birth certificate and suddenly Giacinta became of legal working age. She took a job at a carpet store in downtown Yonkers.

Typically, Italian immigrants Americanized their names shortly after they set foot on American soil. They believed this would help them blend into American society. There was nothing glamorous about being Italian at the time, so certain concessions were in order. Although their names changed, they continued traditions that they held dear, like making wine, pasta and sausage from scratch.

Sometime after my grandmother and the girls arrived in New York, my grandfather injured his back and could no longer work in construction. The shock was immense. My grandmother was frightened. "You insisted we come to America, so now what are we going to do? We can't grow food and soon we won't have any money left to buy it!" my grandmother shouted.

My grandfather's relentless optimism did not let my grandmother's comment ruin his day. He felt confident that by asking around, he would find another way of making a living. Serendipitously, he learned that the small general store on the ground floor of their apartment building had opened up for new management. My grandfather loved working with people and thought that renting the general store would be a good opportunity for the family. My grandmother was hesitant at first and was not sure they could succeed in running a business. They didn't have enough money and she was uncomfortable with borrowing.

Nevertheless, they went ahead with the plan since they didn't have any other options. Immigrants didn't have access to bank loans for starting a business. So, like other people in their position, my grandfather borrowed from family and friends until he had enough to take over the general store.

Once their new venture was in full operation, there were plenty of chores to keep the entire family busy. The deli was a great gathering spot for all the locals. My grandfather loved socializing and making small talk and he enjoyed a good party. My grandmother also enjoyed company and they both loved to cook, so they made a good team.

In November 1916, a fourth child was born, a boy they named Fedele. His American name was Freddy. My grandfather thought he had won the lottery—a boy at last! While the going was good, they added another, a baby girl named Rosa, my mother, born in November 1917. Pietro and Petronilla gave birth to two more children in America: Nicola (Nic) in 1919 and Domenico (Dominic) in 1921. There would be eight children altogether, three boys and five girls, some born in Yonkers, and some in Southern Italy.

My grandmother was getting somewhat used to the American culture, but worried constantly about the future of her daughters. "How are we going to provide a dowry for all of them?" she often asked her husband. "It's too early to worry about such things," he said.

Over the years the store was successful, and along with the money earned by their working children, and the cash that came from renting a spare bedroom to single Italian immigrants, there was enough for the family to live on and even to put some money aside.

CHAPTER 7

A MOMENTOUS DECISION

As time passed, my grandparents' eldest daughter, Jenny (Giacinta), now 17, had moved on from her first job and was working in a dress factory where she learned to make beaded evening gowns.

"This is the perfect job for you. You can make your own wedding dress when the time comes," opined her ever-practical mother. "You can even make wedding dresses for your younger sisters."

Jenny looked forward to her wedding day, like every young lady her age. Eligible bachelors were already noticing her, and of course, her parents' and younger sisters' watchful eyes were on her every move. At that time, an Italian courtship was carried on in secret until the couple was ready to make it official and announce it to their parents. It was considered particularly disrespectful to both families for a couple to be seen in public prior to the official announcement. For some couples, this status could go on for years, especially if the woman had an older, unmarried sister. Luckily for Jenny, this was not the case; she was the oldest daughter.

The fine young man who won the battle for Jenny's heart was Jimmy (Vincenzo) Sarubbi, a WWI veteran and immigrant, also from Southern Italy. In fact, he was from the very same farm community as Jenny's family. He had entered the United States as a young teenager and became an American citizen while serving in the United States Army. During the war, Jimmy was wounded when a shell exploded next to him. The story goes that he was at first overlooked in the rubble. But, fortunately, he was saved thanks to the keen eye of one of his comrades who noticed a speck of a soldier's uniform and dug him out. His injuries left him with a permanent limp.

In the Cosentino family, a little turmoil was brewing. There was talk of returning to Italy. It's not clear who the instigator of that idea was. Some say my grandfather's physician had told them the climate in Italy would be better for my grandfather's health. Others claimed that my grandmother never got used to living in America and always wished to return home.

Whatever the reason or reasons, the Cosentinos decided that they had saved up enough money to return to Italy, have a good life, and reunite with the rest of the family. Jenny was unfazed by these discussions, because she planned to marry Jimmy and stay in America.

When Jimmy approached my grandfather and asked permission to marry Jenny, he expected to receive unconditional approval. After all, not only was he already employed, but he was from the same town as the Cosentinos. He thought the Cosentinos would be happy to welcome him into their family.

My grandfather's response, however, came as a disappointing surprise. "I'm sure you would be an excellent husband for Jenny, but before we discuss marriage there is something you should know. I'm thinking of returning to Italy with the whole family," my grandfather said. Jimmy was stunned.

"Really! Why are you thinking of doing that? Don't you like it here?" Jimmy asked.

"Yes, I do like it here but it's a little more complicated than that," my grandfather replied.

Jimmy was trying to understand. Jenny's father had worked so hard to bring the family here and now he wanted to uproot the family again and go back to Italy? Why would he possibly want to do that? Some immigrants repatriate because they never succeed in bringing their entire family to America, and others do it because with the money they had earned they could move up the social ladder in Italy, something that would be unattainable in America. The latter is probably the reason my grandfather decided to return to Italy. Here, he would always be an uneducated immigrant. He would have to watch his children grow up in a culture he could barely understand and he would always remain at the bottom of the pile.

"When are you thinking of moving?" Jimmy asked.

"Not for a while yet, but if we do the whole family is coming with me, including Jenny," replied my grandfather.

"Does that mean that I can't marry Jenny?"

"No, it doesn't," said my grandfather, "but it means you would have to come to Italy with us and marry Jenny there with the rest of the family present."

As long as he could marry Jenny, Jimmy was willing to accept the conditions. He knew that in their culture, the bride's father would always have the last word until his daughter was married.

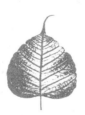

CHAPTER 8

A DREAM MEETS REALITY

Italy ended World War I on the side of the winners along with the United States, Great Britain, France, and Russia. Like all countries involved in World War I, Italy suffered immense loss, including almost two million people dead, wounded, or crippled for life. Economic problems were rampant and a high percentage of the population was living below the poverty line, especially in the south of Italy.

If one reads history books, the situation becomes clear. Serious problems associated with labor unions, riots, strikes, and deflation tore at the social fabric of the country. Military defectors, church involvement, and land re-distribution issues also complicated life after the war. In this climate, the Italian government was unable to establish order. As a consequence, the elections of 1919 saw the Socialist Party and the Italian People's Party come to power.

Italy would not prosper for many, many years, in fact, not for decades. But my grandfather, then living in New York with his wife and seven children, felt certain he had saved enough money to deal with any financial turmoil that might arise. Besides, they already owned land where they had grown up. They believed they would not need much money to live in a farm community without electricity, running water, or infrastructure.

After all, there was plenty of wood for heating, lots of fresh water in the creek right by the house, and no utility bills to pay. They would be able to grow their own food, raise barnyard animals like chickens and rabbits to eat, and larger farm animals to eat or sell for cash when needed. What could be better?

No doubt he was also convinced that after the war the Italian government would rebuild the country and eventually bring roads, running water, and electricity, even into the poor region of Basilicata where they were going to live. They would be able to enjoy the same comforts they now had in America, plus be with family.

My grandfather read the newspapers and listened to the Italian broadcasts on the radio on a regular basis, but unfortunately he was a bit of a dreamer and not fully aware as to what was really going on in Italy. He also could not have predicted the increasing political and social turmoil that would follow the war. He didn't know that hunger was rampant in post-war Italy, which meant farmers were required to share their crops through government programs or be fined.

"There might not be any electricity for now, but the air is clean, the water is fresh," my grandfather would have said.

"We will be with family and that is more important than anything else," my grandmother surely told her children. "You can go to school or learn a trade, just like here."

"And we will probably be able to afford household help," my grandfather added.

His older children were not excited about leaving their life in New York, the place they now called home. But with both parents making convincing arguments about repatriating, they eventually accepted the idea.

Confident that he had a plan that would work, the family packed up everything they could, including Petronilla's favorite punch bowl with 12 cups that hung around the edge. They were proud to take America with them. In the summer of 1921, the Cosentinos boarded a ship in New York harbor bound for Italy. They spent a fairly uneventful month at sea. The waters were smooth and no one got seasick.

As the ship approached the port of Naples, the first news-worthy information that circulated amongst the passengers was that Italy's beloved tenor, Enrico Caruso, had died. This was heartbreaking for many, because this world-renowned tenor was a hero for all Italians, particularly emigrants living in distant lands. Through his beautiful and emotionally stirring interpretation of many Neapolitan songs and well known arias, Caruso was able to bring comfort to their souls during difficult times when they were most homesick. My grandparents had often listened to his music with friends and neighbors throughout their years in America.

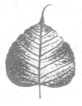

CHAPTER 9

THE "AMERICAN FAMILY" RETURNS

Once in Naples, the Cosentinos were greeted by family members who helped them complete the laborious journey home. The trip that now takes less than two hours by car then took two days by bus, train, mules, and donkeys. The closer they got to the farm, the entourage grew in number as more and more family and friends joined in.

The farm community had been anticipating and preparing for the American family's arrival for weeks and weeks. It was so unusual for people to repatriate that the Cosentinos return seemed like a miracle. Everyone was bustling in all directions, preparing for the festivities and bubbling with, "reunion anxiety." After all, this was the return of people who had seen the world and whom they never thought they would see again! But, how would the old farm look to the Cosentinos now?

The day the Cosentino family of nine arrived at the farm has been remembered by the locals in Seluci as a divine emotional moment. The tears of joy and long embraces lasted forever. They had seven years of catching up to do. Jenny's fiancé, Jimmy, was also from this area, so there were two families celebrating the return of loved ones they had never expected to see again.

In those days, the only way to share news was through a telegram or a letter. As a result, a lot of family experience just went unreported. It would take weeks before the Cosentinos would fall into the ordinary routine of the village. The "American family," as they were called now, settled in their maternal grandmother's house with plans to build a large extension, in accordance with my grandfather's plan. This primitive lifestyle in the rugged hills of Basilicata was now their future.

CHAPTER 10

LIFE ON THE FARM

The lives of almost everyone in the farm community revolved around the agricultural calendar. They seeded the fields in the spring and harvested throughout the summer and fall. People were used to being flexible, because the calendar was only as reliable as the weather; nature always had the last word. In order to survive in this region, each nuclear family had to own some land and have good crops every year. Depending upon the size of the family, some families would send older children to work as paid day labor on other farms to help make ends meet.

The Cosentinos had arrived back in Basilicata not long before the wheat harvest that would take place in the month of July. Only Jenny and her parents had clear memories of how much work was required on a farm that was completely non-mechanized. The transition to a primitive lifestyle based on hard physical labor would prove difficult for the entire family.

Typical days on the farm started very early with the sound of the rooster crowing. "When you hear the rooster singing, it means that it's time to get up, even if it's still dark out," Petronilla would remind her children at bedtime. So many tasks were required in the home just to begin the day, everyone was eager to get up and get started so they wouldn't fall behind.

The first meal of the day consisted of polenta with a simple sprinkle of cheese or a tomato sauce with sausage, depending on what was available. However, in order to make that meal, first they had to start a fire in the fireplace, then boil the water in a kettle on a tripod, and then slowly add the cornmeal flour while stirring constantly to avoid lumps.

While this task of making polenta was usually in the hands of the adult women, the men would take care of the large farm animals, feeding them, and cleaning their stalls. The children would carry water from the spring to the house, looking after their younger siblings, and feeding the small farm animals such as chickens and rabbits. When the polenta was ready, one of the family members would step outside and with a loud yodel, announce that the first meal of the day was ready.

Immediately after eating, everyone would again scatter around the farm to attend to whatever needed doing that day, such as taking the animals out to pasture, mending fences, gathering food from the vegetable garden, cleaning the house, going to the river to do laundry, and hanging clothes to dry on a line.

Family bonds in the farm community were very strong. It was a given that from a very young age, children would be included in most family activities. Depending on each family's resources, these responsibilities were sometimes very heavy. But, the children knew that they were part of their family's success and they took great joy in imitating whatever the adults were doing.

On bread-making days, mothers gave their children their own pieces of dough to play with, or to make miniature pizzas, dolls, or figurines. They were allowed to bake their creations once the wood-burning brick oven was ready. Except for cold winter days, children spent most of their time outdoors climbing trees, running, picking fruit, carving portraits out of squashes, and playing with small farm animals.

One of the chores that they really enjoyed was delivering verbal messages, good or bad, to nearby families. If this message needed to go beyond the nearby family, then a child from that household would relay the message forward. The parents gave the children strict instructions to deliver the messages accurately and politely. They also reminded them to make a quick getaway and not to stand around waiting for a reward, "like a wilted cucumber." Traditionally, recipients of a message always rewarded the child with a hard candy, a small coin, or a few Jordan almonds. Children rarely had a chance to enjoy sweets, so it was very hard for them to turn down candy. The grown-ups understood this, so they would sometimes follow the child all the way home if they had to, to make sure they accepted the treat.

This messenger service was crucial, because it was the only way to communicate with family and neighbors near and far, since there was no postal service, telephone, or other means of communication. It was especially important as the farm community began to organize the various harvests each year. Collective efforts were necessary, because no family had sufficient labor to accomplish this hard work alone.

Jenny and Jimmy, the soon to be newlyweds, participated fully in every harvest that took place in the Seluci area during the summer and fall of 1921. Jenny's teenage sisters, Maria and Feluccia, took turns looking after their four younger siblings, helping the older women prepare the meals of the day, working with the group in the field, or going to the stream to fill the water jugs.

The wheat fields of the Cosentino's farm were first on the schedule that summer. The activities started before dawn. The adults with young children organized themselves so that the children would always be safe and protected during the very long and busy days. One way to keep the youngest babies safe was to place them in wicker bassinets covered with a veil to protect them from flies. Resembling enormous fruits, the baskets hung in shade trees while the adults were working in the fields.

The men cut the wheat by hand using a sickle. The women followed behind the men, gathering up the cut wheat and tying it into bundles. By the end of the first day of this hard labor, everyone noticed the red faces of the Cosentino girls.

"Petronilla, look at your daughters' faces. They're so red. I don't think your girls should work so long in the sun. We're used to it, but they're not," said one of Cosentino relatives.

"They have to get used to working outdoors just like the rest of us. If they are old enough to eat on their own, they are old enough to participate in growing the food that they are going to eat," said Petronilla.

The next day, everyone returned to the field to carry the bundles of wheat to the outdoor threshing floor, a hardened surface that each family maintained year around. Cows pulled the huge threshing stone that crushed the wheat, separating the grain from the straw. Once they accomplished this task, everyone helped bundle up the straw and hand-carry it to the barn to use for feed and other purposes. They then swept up the wheat berries left on the ground and stored them in burlap bags. Harvesting the wheat was very hard work and it went on for days.

When the time was right, with the help of the wind, they separated the wheat from the chaff in a process called winnowing. They flipped the wheat berries over and over using flat baskets. As the chaff loosened and blew away in the wind, the grain fell to the ground. The wheat berries were again gathered up and stored in sacks. Finally, the women would carry the sacks of grain on their heads, or in baskets hanging on both sides of donkeys, to the mill for grinding into flour.

"Well girls, you made it through your first wheat harvest. That wasn't so bad, was it?" said my grandfather to his daughters, jokingly, as they were finishing up the work on the last field.

"My hands are all scratched up, and I'm all sunburned, and all my muscles hurt," Maria complained to their father.

"Don't worry, you'll have a chance to rest before the corn harvest. That one's less work and a lot more fun, you'll see. During the corn harvest there will be a party and dancing every night," he said, attempting to make his daughters feel better.

Jenny reiterated to her sisters what her father had said, but she was secretly rejoicing in the fact that she and Jimmy would be married and returning to America within a few months. This was the only summer she would have to work in the fields.

On the other hand, Maria and Feluccia were distraught at the idea they would be spending every future summer, year after year, working in the wheat fields, bringing in the harvest. What they had initially thought of as a fun activity, they now realized was also very hard physical labor. They envied their three younger siblings, Fedele, Dominico, and my mother Rosina, all under five years of age, who were still young enough to be pampered and not expected to work.

That night, my grandfather Pietro said to Petronilla, "We made it through our first harvest back in Italy. It was more work than I remembered, but now we have enough flour to make bread for at least a year. If we have bread we have everything."

"And if we are blessed with good health, then that is more than everything," Petronilla added.

With the wheat harvest behind them, the families of the Seluci community and beyond were happy to return to their usual long days of farm work. In addition to the regular tasks of tending the animals and watering the crops, at this time of year tomatoes ripening on the vine needed to be picked, canned, or dried, plus, beans to pick, dry, and shell, and squashes to gather, slice, de-seed, and dry.

September came around quickly and the corn was ripe. Everyone looked forward to the corn harvest because it was accomplished in steps over several days, so there was always enough time and energy left over to have a dancing party at the end of each day.

Men and women worked side-by-side cutting the stalks with a sickle and tying them in bundles. They would firmly stack the bundles together to dry in a vertical position while still in the field. Once the corn was dry enough, the largest room of the house was cleared out completely. They brought all the corn inside and the shucking party would start.

Shucking the corn was a tedious process that didn't take much concentration, so it was an opportunity to tell funny jokes, tease each other, and race to finish one's pile first. These shucking parties were a perfect time for the single men and women to size each other up, talk, and flirt. It was during the corn harvest, amidst the bright colors of early fall, that many love stories sparked. The elders kept a close eye on every glance, every gesture, and every smile. It would become valuable material for the gossip corner during the upcoming long days of winter.

After shucking the corn, they arranged the cobs on blankets in the sun to dry some more. They stuffed the husks into burlap bags and stored them in the barn. Once the ears of corn were nice and dry, they sorted them into piles. Only the highest quality ears would go in the pile for human consumption.

The next step in the process was to remove the kernels from the dried ears. To accomplish this task, they would cover the floor with a specially woven rag rug and spread the ears of corn over it. Each man, woman, and child would use a stick to pound the ears until all the kernels had fallen off the cobs. The bare cobs would be put aside for feed and they would then lift the rug around the perimeter to gather the kernels into the center. They shoveled the kernels into burlap bags that they would later take to the mill to grind into corn flour. Once they transported the sacks of flour back into their homes, the women sifted the flour, filling linen sacks with only the finest part for later use to make polenta. They saved the corn bran for feeding the pigs and chickens.

After each of the major steps in processing of the corn crop, a dance party would start when one of the accordion players would play a few chords of the *tarantella*, making his way to the dance floor. He would be followed by all of the men who would wave to the ladies to join in. Everyone learned this traditional dance from the time they could walk, so the children joined in as well.

They continued dancing mazurkas, waltzes, and many other ballroom dances all evening. Occasionally, somebody passed around a small glass of wine along with homemade pretzels. After each party, people walked home under the moonlight or using oil lamps to light their way. The Cosentino teenagers began to feel revitalized. They were able to see that young men their age were fun to be with. They were great dancers, they had beautiful smiles, they told funny jokes, and above all, they were always gentlemen.

Nature had saved the best for last. The occasional slight chill in the air would be a sweet reminder that the grapes were ripening and would soon be ready to pick and turn into wine. Each family grew enough grapes to make at least one or two barrels of wine every year. My grandfather, who loved his wine with every meal, had been looking forward to this particular harvest since before the family left America. Being able to spend time with his siblings, cousins, and friends making wine once again would be the best that life had to offer.

The grape harvest usually took place toward the end of September or early October. They would collect the grapes in large wicker baskets and transfer them into a stomping barrel. The bottom was slanted enough so the juice would automatically flow out through a hole near the base and into a wooden pitcher. They would then pour the juice into an aging barrel using a wooden funnel. They would store the barrels of new wine in the cellar or designated room, not to be disturbed until the 8th of December, the Feast of the Solemnity of the Immaculate Conception, the official beginning of the Christmas season, and the day for tasting the new wine. With the attics and storage rooms well stocked, people in this small community felt reassured that they could survive for at least another annual cycle of harvests.

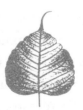

CHAPTER 11

JENNY AND JIMMY'S WEDDING

The month of November was approaching and the Cosentino family began focusing on Jenny and Jimmy's wedding which would precede their permanent departure to America. Their respective parents and siblings had been too busy with farm work to focus on this bittersweet event. The wedding and departure would change the dynamics of the Cosentino and Sarubi families forever. There would be some very sad days ahead.

Jenny (born in 1901) was the oldest of the Cosentino's daughters, while my mother, Rosina, was at that time the youngest daughter. The wedding was scheduled for November 1921, because Jenny and Jimmy's six-month visas would soon expire.

The glorious wedding gown Jenny had brought from America waited to be unpacked. The young woman had labored nearly every night for a year over the elaborate beadwork creation. She had applied the same painstaking effort and artistry that defined her workday at the dress factory in America, but with a heady infusion of love and hope. Once completed, this dress was a one-of-a-kind, glorious work of art. Jenny was going to look like a princess from another world, a beauty that until then had only existed in imagination.

In the farm community, however, it was not customary for the bride to wear a long, fancy, white gown at her wedding. As soon as Jenny's mother-in-law-to-be heard rumors about the dress, holy hell broke loose. Turmoil ruled in the farm community. Everyone took a side in favor of, or against, Jenny wearing the beautiful dress.

"Everybody's poor here. It's out of place and out of tradition to wear such a dress. Perhaps in a big city but not here!" somebody would say.

"It's her wedding. Let her wear what she wants," someone else would chime in.

"If she wears that big fancy dress, she will be the talk of the community. People will gossip about it forever and we'll never hear the end of it. It's better to honor tradition," Jimmy's mother insisted.

Lucky for the mother-in-law, members of the Cosentino family were well-mannered and had a great sense of humor. Poised and sensitive to the local traditions, eager to restore joy and harmony in the community, the soon-to-be newlyweds accepted the wishes of the mother-in-law and removed Jenny's beaded creation from their wedding plans. According to my sources, the famous wedding dress was donated to the local church.

When I first heard the story I was sad and furious. I would have gladly said a thing or two to the mother-in-law. I would have thrown a fit, slammed some doors, and worn my wedding dress in the end. Today, as I reflect on the story, I think how grand and selfless of my aunt Jenny and of my grandmother to accommodate the local traditions in spite of what must have been an enormous disappointment.

The wedding turned out to be in keeping with regional traditions. The ceremony itself was modest, but the food and accordion music that followed made the day special. Immediately after the wedding, the young couple made their rounds, saying their final and tearful goodbyes to everyone in the Seluci area. This stirred up familiar and painful feelings of loss, because they all knew someone who had emigrated, never to return.

Southern Italy's economic situation was disastrous. With unemployment rates sky-high, there was no way to make a living, and anybody who could find a way to escape this dire situation was leaving for faraway lands. There they hoped to find some kind of work that would allow them to send money home to support their starving families.

On the day of departure, before dawn, the family entourage, some on foot, some on horseback, or on mule, or donkey, escorted Jenny and

Jimmy to the distant edge of the farm. They walked in silence because it was too difficult to speak. With every step she took, Petronilla agonized about what was to come. She wanted time to stand still, to stretch out each moment as long as possible.

She now realized what her own parents had experienced when she moved to join her husband in New York. Petronilla asked herself, how do you say goodbye to one of your children forever? The only thing that gave her any peace of mind was the knowledge that Jenny and Jimmy were returning to the same neighborhood where they had all previously lived in New York. The Cosentinos had established some strong friendships in Yonkers, New York, and she knew they were going to be surrounded by a community much like the one they were leaving behind.

When that final dreadful moment came, Petronilla held her daughter in her arms and wept. "Goodbye my dear daughter. Be well and take care of yourself. I know that God will bless you with many beautiful, healthy children. And if we live honest lives and pray to God, hopefully we will see each other again in Heaven."

Jenny was speechless. Until this moment she had not fully understood the consequences of her decision to marry and go back to America without her family. We will never see our parents again, and our children will grow up without the love and support of their grandparents, she thought to herself as tears fell from her eyes.

Jimmy and Jenny completed the trip to the port of Naples only with their fathers. There, they boarded the ship that would take them across the Atlantic and back to America.

CHAPTER 12

HOLIDAY TRADITIONS

The Cosentinos spent their first winter back in Italy in the company of their extended family members; with the very people whom they had talked about, but couldn't see, when they were living in America. The days were short and the family spent a great deal of time around the fireplace, trying to keep warm just like all the families in the area.

During the winter months, men would go away for weeks at a time to work on licorice farms, harvesting the licorice root. Petronilla and the other women would stay home and catch up on chores they had put aside during the busier months: mending, sewing, knitting, weaving, cooking, taking care of the children, and keeping the hogs and other farm animals fed. No matter how busy they were, these women made time to embroider sheets and pillowcases that would eventually be part of their daughters' dowries.

By Christmas Eve, all the men who had gone away to work had returned home. They were all devout Catholics and the families celebrated Christmas the same way every year.

On Christmas Eve, Petronilla, like all the other housewives, busied herself preparing the special Christmas meal. Tradition called for *baccala*, a salt-preserved cod that was reconstituted by soaking it in water for forty-eight hours and then poaching it in tomato sauce. Unlike every other day of the year, *baccala* was served with store-bought pasta — everyone agreed that *baccala* tasted better with store-bought spaghetti or linguine.

After dinner, weather permitting, those who could would walk together for over an hour to the nearest church to attend midnight Mass, singing Christmas carols all the way. Everyone looked forward to this special event and felt deep sadness if they weren't able to attend.

On Christmas Day, the meal consisted of meat sauce made mostly from stewed rabbit or other farm animals and handmade pasta. Relatives would gather and share the meal. No gifts were exchanged. Holiday treats were simple, but delicious. Everyone's favorite was the *chiulini*, a ravioli-shaped pastry often stuffed with chestnut or chickpea puree, flavored with cocoa, sugar or honey, and cinnamon, and then baked to a golden brown in the wood oven.

The last celebration of the holiday season was the Epiphany. On Epiphany Eve all the children hung their stockings by the fireplace before they went to bed hoping that "La Befana," an old lady flying on a broomstick, would come down the chimney and leave candy for them and not coal. Although the parents often threatened them with coal, "La Befana" always left them candy.

The main activity that punctuated the winter months was the slaughtering of the hog in late January. It was an opportunity to get together with family and neighbors to accomplish this very important task as a team. Except for an occasional chicken, rabbit, or goat killed for some exceptional reason, the hog was the main source of meat that people used to flavor or accompany dishes year-round. Seeing all the newly preserved meat gave everyone a sense of comfort knowing that if they rationed correctly, they would have food available for the upcoming year.

The Cosentinos and all the other families would choose a date to slaughter their hog which they had spent a whole year fattening up. Only certain people with proven experience were allowed to perform the actual slaughter. Once they prepped the animal, the main artery had to be punctured accurately and quickly; it was considered bad luck to let the animal suffer for longer than necessary.

They drained the blood, shaved the pig, removed the skin, and butchered the animal. Everyone worked swiftly and diligently, handling the meat properly to avoid spoilage. They put the prosciuttos in brine. They ground and seasoned the meat to make sausage and salami, stuffed it into the proper intestine casings and then hung them where there was proper ventilation for drying and curing.

They also preserved some of the fresh sausage in lard to avoid oxidization. A family was able to pull a piece of sausage out of the lard at a moment's notice and cook it in a frying pan or directly on the flame of the fireplace. It required a lot of willpower during long winter nights by the fire not to raid the sausage pot, because sausage cooked on the open flame was everyone's favorite treat.

Every last scrap of the hog was used purposefully, including the blood. The women strained the blood and then added it to precooked rice and breadcrumbs flavored with chocolate, honey, cinnamon, and lots of raisins. They would line pots or pans with pastry dough, pour in the mixture and top it with a final layer of pastry. They would then bake it slowly in the brick wood-oven until the crusts were a beautiful, rich golden brown. This wonderful treat was called *sanguinaccio* and it was eaten at room temperature the next day. I remember as a child not sleeping at night when I knew that there was *sanguinaccio* waiting for me in the morning.

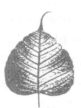

CHAPTER 13

NEWS FROM AMERICA

The Cosentinos had been waiting anxiously to receive their first letter from Jenny and Jimmy. It finally arrived shortly after the slaughtering of the hogs and brought much joy to the immediate and extended family.

In their letter, Jenny and Jimmy wrote about the warm welcome they received from everyone upon their return to America. They had settled in a house on Beech Street, in the same neighborhood where they had lived before they married. Beech Street was a cul-de-sac and became almost like a family compound. All the children played in the street safely. When the men returned from work every day, they would call out to the entire neighborhood and were welcomed home as part of a large, loving family.

On Beech Street there was never a dull moment and it even became like a smaller version of the farm community in Italy. Everyone got along and helped each other with taking care of children, cooking, errands, and other aspects of daily life.

Summer evenings were particularly magnificent on Beech Street. To avoid the indoor heat, people gathered in backyards where they enjoyed a slice of cold watermelon, or a dish of ice cream, or sipped a whisky and soda. Children loved circulating from one yard to another to socialize and enjoy the different treats.

Jenny and Jimmy raised five children on Beech Street. Their home became the locus of settlement for many family members. They witnessed many immigrants come and go throughout the years. In the 1950s they welcomed Jenny's younger siblings, Fidele and Dominico, and their families. In the mid-1960s they welcomed my family. Unfortunately, Jenny and Jimmy were never able to return to Basilicata until 51 years later, long after both sets of parents were gone.

CHAPTER 14

HARD TIMES, NEW LIFE

The financial devastation in Italy following WWI had a profound impact on everyone. Naively, my grandfather had returned to Italy, never imagining the profound impact the aftermath of the war would have on his family. When they returned from America, the exchange rate from the US dollar to the Italian *lira* was very favorable, and my grandfather believed he was financially safe for the foreseeable future.

However, the money that he had saved while in America didn't go nearly as far as he thought it would. Try as he might, my grandfather was unable to buy more land or build the house of his dreams. Instead, he and my grandmother and all of their children, continued living in a small add-on to the original family home.

In addition to buying land, Pietro Cosentino had planned to send all of his children to school through at least fifth grade, something only families with means could afford to do. Unfortunately, the school system in rural Seluci, where my grandparents lived, was very minimal. Laws enacted in 1859 and 1877 required compulsory primary education for all children throughout the country. However, these laws did not take effect in Basilicata until decades after my grandfather returned to Italy.

In the 1920s illiteracy was still close to 80 percent. Children attended classes in a one-room schoolhouse just two hours per day, through third grade for the boys and first grade for the girls. The thinking was that as future housewives, girls didn't need much schooling. Boys, however, needed to have some preparation for the military draft.

Unfortunately, the conditions in Italy meant that none of my grandfather's big plans worked out. It also meant that my mother was unable to get the education she would have received if the family had stayed in New York. That reality haunted my mother throughout her life.

While Jenny and Jimmy were raising their young family in Yonkers, New York, her parents, Pietro and Petronilla, had their eighth and last child, Antonietta, in 1927. In rural Basilicata, children like Antonietta were born at home with the assistance of midwives and the female relatives of the expectant mother. The common practice was that the grandparents, aunts, uncles, and neighbors would take the youngest children into their homes during this time.

After giving birth, the new mother would eat chicken soup, stewed rabbit, and other delectable dishes freshly prepared and provided just for her by family and friends. Elder women in the community determined when the new mother was "good and ready" to gradually resume her usual activities.

The birth of Antonietta greatly increased the family chores. Laundry was one of the hardest tasks to accomplish. Petronilla and her daughters would walk to the river's edge once or twice a week to do laundry. They would soak each item in the water, lay it on a rock and rub it with a big cake of soap, scrub it repeatedly on the rock, and then rinse it out in the river. They carried the laundry both ways in wicker baskets balanced on their heads. Once home they would hang each item on outdoor clotheslines, but if the weather didn't permit, they would string ropes around the whole house creating a wonderful maze of laundry for children playing hide and seek.

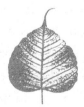

CHAPTER 15

"MY COUNTRY DOESN'T LOVE ME"

Time went on as it always does and members of the Cosentino family were always busy trying to keep up with farm chores, day after day, season after season. By the early 1930s the second oldest Cosentino daughter, Maria, had married. The third daughter, Feluccia, soon did the same. My mother, a teenager by then, was just starting to make heads turn.

The post-World War I years did not bring much economic relief to the already impoverished Southern regions of Italy. The Cosentino family still did not own much land and struggled to produce enough food to eat. Fascism under Mussolini was not delivering everything it had promised. Disillusionment was settling in amongst all Italians.

Every morning, my grandfather rose early, like all farmers. He would step outside, ready to start the day. On his way to the barn where he kept his tools, he would turn his head toward the sunrise and stop.

"Every day that the sun rises, I will regret leaving America. Damn the devil who tempted me to leave. I love my country, but my country doesn't love me. All these years have passed since we came back and still nothing is mechanized on our farms; there's no electricity, no running water! Nothing has improved. I'm working like a mule every day to just to put enough food on the table so my family doesn't go hungry."

This harsh reality convinced him the only solution was to return to America. He would have to swallow his pride and find a way to convince his wife to relocate again without getting his head chopped off. Neither of them wanted to admit they had had a role in making the catastrophic decision to bring the family back to Italy.

He began by creating scenarios while playing with his youngest daughter, little Antonietta, who was about five at that time. He would talk about how nice it would be for her to grow up in America, where she could go to school, learn to speak English, and become a secretary or a teacher.

"You would wear a business suit and gloves to work. And you would one day perhaps learn to drive a car and even own one. In America anything is possible. Besides, you have an older sister who already lives there. She has children your age, and would love for us all to be together again," he would tell her.

He would show his little girl pictures of her sister Jenny and her family in New York. Antonietta was very intrigued. One night after dinner, Antonietta asked her mother, "When are we going to go back to America?"

"What do you know about America?" Petronilla asked as she cleared the table. "Is your father putting ideas in your head?"

Little by little, my grandfather managed, through his crafty discussions with his granddaughter, to insert his wish into my grandmother's head and soon enough, it sounded like it was her own idea. It didn't take long before the entire family was dreaming about returning to America.

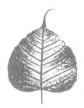

CHAPTER 16

AN UNSPEAKABLE TRAGEDY

During the summer of 1933, Pietro and Petronilla prepared for the wheat harvest, as they did every year. They set the date to begin and announced it to the extended family and friends who usually helped them. The Cosentinos never had trouble finding extra hands, because they were well liked and were known for throwing great parties after a hard day of work. Early in the morning when all the help arrived, the Cosentinos served breakfast in the field. This consisted of their homemade prosciutto, salami, cheese, and bread. Around 11 o'clock, they presented another round of food; then the main meal was served around 2 p.m.

My grandmother would usually make a rabbit stew in tomato sauce to season her homemade tagliatelle or gnocchi. She would pack the entire meal into wide wicker baskets that she and some of the women carried to the field on their heads. They would lower the baskets to the ground and begin unpacking the delicacies. The linen covers were unwrapped allowing the sumptuous aromas to escape. Although everyone was plenty hungry, they continued to work to avoid looking impolite. Finally, after being urged to stop and come to eat, they would gather in the shade of a big tree. While they ate, they told funny stories and jokes, teased each other, and enjoyed a long siesta afterward. They resumed working around 4:30 and stopped at sundown.

The wheat harvest was a time of exuberance. It was a great opportunity for young men and women to get to know each other, to assess who was who and what was what. Children had the time of their lives playing, running around, and climbing trees with other children their age.

One harvest morning, after the crew had finished their first breakfast, my grandmother busied herself in the kitchen as usual, getting the big meal started. My mother, then age sixteen, went to the field to deliver the late-morning snack. When she came back to the house, she and Petronilla made several trips to the water source to fill up the ten-gallon kettle to boil the water for cooking the homemade pasta. Once the pasta was cooked, two people carefully removed the kettle from the tripod on the fireplace and set the kettle on the floor in order to scoop up the pasta to mix with the sauce in large pasta bowls. While this operation was taking place, children were chased out of the kitchen for obvious reasons.

Little Antonietta was outside jumping about like a bunny with an empty stomach waiting for lunch. At one point, she stepped into the kitchen to announce how hungry she was. "Stay away from the kitchen!" one of the women shouted. "Stay away from the hot kettle!" shouted Petronilla.

But, unfortunately for Antonietta, it was already too late. She was already skipping around the kitchen like a carefree six-year old and got too close to the kettle. Before anyone could catch her she tripped and fell into the still boiling water with everything but her head and feet submerged.

The unimaginable had happened and now pandemonium followed. The frantic women pulled her out of the boiling kettle instantly, but she was in shock from the pain. My mother ran to the field to alert everyone. Work stopped immediately and they all ran to the house to provide help. They tried giving her some sugared water to drink, the only remedy they had available to give children when all else failed. Hugging, cuddling, rocking, singing was to no avail. Antonietta's skin had been severely scalded and no amount of cuddling, praying, or sugared water could ease her pain.

My grandfather moved like lightning. Within minutes, he had the mule saddled up and in front of the house, ready to rush his little girl to the nearest town to see a doctor. He immediately discovered that Antonietta was in too much pain to tolerate the movements of the mule. He took his little girl in his arms and started the two-and-half mile journey to reach the nearest town on foot. One of the male relatives jumped on the mule and galloped ahead to locate the only doctor in the area and make sure that he was waiting for my grandfather once he arrived.

The doctor did his best with what he had available. He gave a treatment for my grandparents to follow and sent them back home.

Not too many details are available to me about this tragedy because whenever my mother tried to talk about it, she would break down and was unable to continue with the story. My grandmother managed to keep a strong face around her injured little girl, but my grandfather couldn't. Whenever he looked at her, his eyes would fill with tears and he had to look away. When Antonietta saw her father in such pain, she would say to him, "Don't cry daddy. I'm not going to die, don't cry."

A few days later, six-year-old Antonietta did die. When the Cosentinos buried their youngest child, they also buried any notion that they would ever go to America and abandon her grave. In New York, when Jenny received the news that she had lost her younger sister, the little girl that she had never even met, she was devastated that she couldn't be with her parents to provide them some comfort. Now that she was raising her own children, she knew what an unspeakable tragedy it would be to lose a child.

The months following Antonietta's death were filled with despair and overwhelming guilt for the Cosentinos. They tortured themselves talking about a million "what-ifs." The only thought that gave them any relief was knowing that little Antonietta had been baptized and died while still sinless—therefore she had been automatically admitted to the kingdom of Heaven and she was already an angel looking over them.

CHAPTER 17

A CHARISMATIC LEADER ARISES

Italy had unified as a country in 1861. As a young country it was still not economically and politically stable, thus unable to withstand the colossal turmoil that followed World War I. A record number of Italians, particularly from the south, were forced to migrate to foreign lands, settling for whatever work they could find to avoid starvation.

A young charismatic politician took advantage of this dire situation and emerged from the rubble with a promising message. He told the population he could bring about a brighter future for all Italians if they would help him rise to power. He attracted millions and millions of desperate citizens to his political rallies which created unprecedented cohesive energy among the people. It was through these electrifying events that Italy became a dictatorship in 1925.

Italians rejoiced, convinced that the future looked bright and that the worst part of their lives would soon be over. Rumors spread among farmers in rural areas that occasionally a well-dressed gentleman was seen talking to people in farm communities. He would ask farmers what improvements they would like to see implemented immediately. They would later discover that this gentleman was in fact Benito Mussolini traveling in disguise, wanting to talk directly to the poorest people in Italy. Whether this information was a rumor or a reality, it was certainly intoxicating. It created a massive following, particularly among the poor and the uneducated.

Mussolini quickly put in place a massive infrastructure program. Communities began seeing schools, roads, and rail systems being built. Public transportation increased and was running more efficiently. As a result of these improvements Italians felt encouraged and optimistic. But on the international level discord was brewing, slowly paving the way for the start of World War II in September of 1939.

CHAPTER 18

A WARTIME WEDDING

My parents, Rosina and Raffaele Cantisani, met during a bean shelling party in 1935. At the time my mother was still mourning a relationship that her father had forced her to end. My father was smitten with my mother. He was ready to ask my grandfather for her hand in marriage. In fact, he hoped they could be wed before he was called to mandatory service in the Italian army. My mother liked him and knew who he was, but wasn't yet ready for a marriage proposal. Less than a year later he was called to service. Their courtship continued from afar.

When my father returned from service in 1938, my mother gave him permission to ask her father for her hand in marriage. Grandfather gave them his blessing and they scheduled their wedding for the spring of 1939. They settled in the Cerasia district, several miles from her parents' farm in Seluci. The tradition was that the groom's father would provide the land for the couple and the bride's family would provide the dowry. The piece of land my father received from his parents was adjacent to the farm where his sister, Teodora, and her family lived.

My parents gave birth to their first child, Biagio, in March of 1940. They were happy to be living right next door to my aunt Teodora, who played a major role in our family as we all grew up.

Within months of Biagio's birth, the community was in turmoil because the war was escalating. The rumor was that every man of enlistment age would be drafted. Every family feared they would not survive without the men. They scrambled to plan for the future, trying to envision growing food and minding a farm and all the animals without any men around.

In just a few months, their fears became reality. Every man of serving age was called to duty, including my father and all of his brothers.

My mother's brothers, all American citizens, were also drafted. At that time there was no limit on the number of men from each family that could be called up. Women of all ages said goodbye to their brothers, sons, husbands, and fathers.

Now more than ever, women bonded together and worked like mules to keep everything going on the farm. Suddenly all the manual labor that had been done as a team fell into the hands of the women, children, and the elderly. There was not one task, big or small, that they did not have to handle.

For my mother, having her sister in-law nearby was a lifesaver during the five years my father was away during the war. Together the two women managed the heavy load that faced them every day in the absence of their men. The daily routine began before sunrise and ended after dark. They turned the soil in the fields with shovels. They irrigated every day at dusk by digging a trench and directing the water where it was needed. They took the animals out to pasture in the morning and led them back to the barn at night. They cleaned the barn and the pigsty and fed the pigs. They fed the rabbits and the chickens and cleaned the coops. In addition to milking the cows, sheep, and goats by hand, they also made the cheese.

They chopped wood then split it and carried it to a sunny area to dry. When it was dry, they carried it into the barn to store for winter. They went to the river to wash clothes then hung them to dry in the sun. They would shear the sheep, spin the wool, weave their own fabric, and knit their own sweaters, socks, and blankets. They made quilts and whatever else they needed in order to survive the cold. They caught birds and hunted for food. They killed chickens, rabbits, lambs; they slaughtered hogs. They dried and canned various foods for their own families and for those who were too old to work. When they were able to can or produce more than they needed, they would sell the extra to have some cash for purchasing things they could not produce such as sugar, salt, and oil.

And of course, they cared for their children. No task could be overlooked. Yes, the women did hold down the fort, and they even managed to put a little bit of money aside. They did all of this with strength and conviction, in spite of knowing that the fathers of their children were fighting a seemingly unending war and could very well not come home.

One of the skills my father made sure my mother learned before he left for war was using a gun, both for hunting and self-defense. Living in such a rural and isolated area, danger could lurk just behind one's house at any moment. The woods of the Basilicata region were notorious for their dense population of wolves. After sundown, everyone prepared for the night as if for sure, they were going to be receiving a visit from hungry wolves. The farm animals were secured in their stalls, the guard dogs wore spiked collars, and every house was equipped with a Dutch door, so that only the top portion needed to be opened to see what was going on outside. Shots could easily be fired, if necessary. The farmhouses were all built at ground level and only one or two rooms in size, so they could be easily defended. Especially after dark, any small sound could cause suspicion and make families feel vulnerable.

My mother spent her long winter evenings knitting by the fire. The little oil lamp did not provide enough light for sewing, mending, or any other similar activity, but knitting was one thing she could do by feel. One evening after putting baby Biagio to sleep, she settled by the fire to knit, as usual. She suddenly heard rustling sounds she thought were wolves getting close to the back of the house. With gun in hand, she opened the window, leaned out, and started shooting, hoping to kill them or scare them away.

Almost simultaneously she heard a yodel, which meant that someone from the community was nearby. She dropped the gun and almost fainted. Oh, I hope I haven't killed anyone, she thought.

"Why didn't you yodel? I could have killed you!" my mother shouted.

"We apologize. We didn't think you could hear us. We were just on our way to the front door to knock," they responded.

At that time it was unusual for anyone to travel after dark, precisely to avoid the possibility of being shot at or eaten by wolves. No matter the time of day, it was customary to announce oneself with a repetitive, loud yodel when approaching a dwelling. Not doing so could be very dangerous because the sounds made while moving through the brush and trees could easily be confused with sounds made by wolves. These travelers had taken a big risk by not yodeling. The incident gave my mother the reputation as a fearless woman who would shoot at any foe who came near her house unannounced.

In addition to the never-ending heavy chores that women tended to every day, they took care of the elders and their own young children when they got sick. They relied mostly on home remedies to cure illnesses. They would consult each other and the elders, especially for advice on guessing the right diagnosis and the proper treatment for it. If the home remedy failed, the situation could quickly turn into a life-threatening emergency. At that point someone would rush to town and bring back a doctor on horseback for a home visit. If no doctor was available, they asked a pharmacist for advice. If neither of these approaches worked, they carried the sick person to the closest town where they hoped they would find help. Prayer was always in their arsenal. Sometimes their prayers were answered and sometimes not.

One day baby Biagio came down with a very high fever. My mother and my Aunt Teodora tried the usual remedies, such as a cold damp cloth on the forehead to bring the fever down. Initially it seemed to work, but the fever came back. One evening, while both women continued their relentless efforts to bring down baby Biagio's life-threatening fever, a relative on his way to a distant town on foot stopped by to spend the night. When this man took a look at baby Biagio, he told my mother, "Rosie, the only option you have is to put your baby in God's hands. I don't think he's going to make it through the night."

When my mother heard those dire words, she became a force of nature. No tears and no prayers! In a flash she bundled up the baby, put him in his wicker bassinet, placed him on her head, and ran out of the house. She galloped like a horse through meadows, streams, and ravines. There were no silvery stars to guide her in the dark night, but the familiar smell of trees and other vegetation reassured her that she was on the right path.

It took her several hours to reach the town. Her mouth was dry from fatigue and running, but when she reached the doctor's house, she pounded on the door and managed to shout, "Help, help, help! Wake up! I need help. I need to see the doctor!"

Finally the housemaid opened the door and said, "I'm sorry, the doctor is sleeping. Can you wait until morning?"

"No, no, no," shouted my mother. "You have to wake him up. My baby is dying!"

The housemaid took one look at the baby and immediately ran to wake up the doctor.

As soon as the doctor examined little Biagio, he administered a shot of the right medication. Within hours baby Biagio's fever came down and he was charming the doctor with his smiles and happy disposition. My mother was so grateful to the doctor for saving her baby. She said to him, "God will bless you in more ways than you can imagine."

"Not with one of these, unfortunately," he said as he held baby Biagio in his arms. He tossed Biagio up and down to make him smile and thought to himself for a moment. Then he turned to my mother and said, "Unfortunately, my wife cannot have children."

My mother paused and said, "I'm very sorry to hear that."

"What if I gave you two million *lire*?" said the doctor sympathetically. He was desperate to have a son of his own and he wanted to convince my mother that giving up her child would be best for everyone. "Your son could grow up in an affluent family and your family would never have to worry about money ever again. You can have more children when your husband returns from the war."

My mother was flabbergasted. She wasn't sure if she was hallucinating from her long run through the night or if she was really hearing those words. The doctor's words were all too real. He was very familiar with the extreme poverty in the south and decided to take a chance. He thought that with money and a little bit of luck, perhaps he could convince a mother from a poverty-stricken family to sell one of her children.

During World War II, for a poor farm family, two million *lire* was an unheard-of fortune. Yes, it definitely would have been like winning the jackpot. Unfortunately for the doctor he didn't know my mother. She would never have considered doing such a thing for any amount of money. Since I've always had an older brother by the name of Biagio, born in March of 1940, I guess he did not get sold, not even for the two million *lire*.

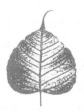

CHAPTER 19

THE WAR COMES HOME

Days passed, weeks went by, seasons made complete cycles, and the war went on. The support that women gave each other provided everyone with the strength to push forward during the lingering years of World War II. No matter how primitive their living conditions or how harsh a tragedy they faced, that sense of belonging made their community strong and precious.

News from the men at war was scarce. But when anyone received a letter, the word spread quickly and everyone gathered around to read it. Few people were literate, so it was often not a close family member who read the letter to the recipient. Bad news was almost always delivered by telegram, so it was usually a joyous occasion when a letter arrived.

My grandfather, Pietro, who had three sons and two sons-in-law fighting in the war, kept himself as informed as he possibly could about everything. He rode his mule to the nearest town of Castelluccio Inferiore on a regular basis to purchase the newspaper and to get the word-of-mouth news from the townspeople. He was well connected and everyone adored him, so it would usually be a long day in town for him. It would take him quite some time before he made all his social rounds, where he was obliged to have at least a glass of wine at every stop.

My mother told me that when my grandfather rode his mule home from town late at night, he would often fall asleep on the way. Luckily, the mule knew the route home, and lucky for my grandfather the mule was always the designated driver. The morning following his day in town, he always read the newspaper from front to back. Everyone in the farm community who was not serving in the war relied on Pietro Cosentino for the latest news.

One fall morning, Pietro sat on a tree stump in front of his house to read the newspaper he had brought home the night before. His salt and pepper hair sparkled in the sunshine. The empty fields all around were quiet and the hills in the distance looked ready for winter. The occasional chirping of a bird and the murmuring of the crisp orange leaves of autumn were the only sounds interrupting the silence around him.

Pietro unfolded his newspaper and began to read. When he reached the list of fallen soldiers, he stopped to cross himself and recited the *Pro, defunctis,* a Latin prayer to honor the dead, a ritual he always followed. Suddenly, he put the paper down and looked away in disbelief. His eyes filled with tears. When he regained his strength, he picked the paper up again and read the list of the fallen soldiers over and over, hoping his eyes had betrayed him. His chest filled with a choking pain. He could hardly breathe as he recognized the name of his son Nicola among the

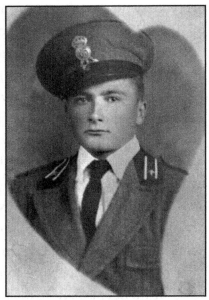

Uncle Nicola in his Italian Army uniform.

dead. The young man had been killed while bringing ammunition to the front line.

"Is this the only way my country knows how to deliver to me the most horrible news a parent can ever receive?" my grandfather asked himself. "My son is dead. Nicola is dead," he sobbed. "My son is dead." He remained alone on the tree stump in front of the house for a long time. He wanted to spare the rest of the family this tragic news for as long as possible.

As he wept, he noticed someone in the distance riding a horse toward him. He quickly recognized a town official coming to deliver the news. My grandfather rose to his feet and walked toward the rider. Once he was able to make eye contact with the official, he held up the newspaper and signaled for him to turn back. The official's condolences were too late.

My grandfather looked around him and everywhere he looked, he saw his son's face. He wished he could go back to not knowing. He wished he could replace his son in death. After all, he had lived a good portion of his life already. His son was only twenty years old. He dreaded having to tell my grandmother that she had lost yet another child. And he would have to tell his other children, the ones near and far, that they had lost their brother, Nicola, to the war.

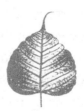

CHAPTER 20

A PRICELESS GESTURE

Jenny (Giacinta), who had been living and raising her five children in Yonkers, New York, was devastated when she received the news of her brother Nicola's death. The last time she had seen him was in 1921, right after she married Jimmy and left Italy to live in America. He had been barely two years old. There wasn't much she could do to console her family from a distance. She wished so much that she could be with them, cry with them, pray with them. She wrote them letters with reassuring words. "Nicola died fighting for the country. Jesus and the Holy Mary will look after him. He is safe. It was God's will."

Whenever she could, she sent a care package to her family filled with clothes for everyone. She would accept donations from her friends at Mount Carmel Church, where people still remembered the Cosentino family very well from when they used to live in Yonkers.

When my grandmother received a package from Jenny and Jimmy, she would wait for everyone in the family to be present before opening the big cardboard box. She would take things out one at a time, smell them, and hold them close to her as though she were hugging her daughter. In every care package Jenny included the latest pictures of her growing children. That always brought a lot of happiness to the family.

When my grandmother looked at the pictures, her eyes would immediately fill with tears of mixed joy and melancholy. She wished that one day she could meet her grandchildren and see her daughter again. But deep inside she knew that was only a wish. Travel was extremely expensive. Families of modest means never traveled anywhere unless it was for work or to relocate permanently.

Sending care packages became a tradition that still lives on in my family. There is something magical about receiving a care package, particularly if it is unexpected. It is a priceless gesture.

I remember receiving packages from my mother for every special occasion throughout my entire adult life, even if I planned to join the family for the holiday. She honored this tradition for as long as she could. My father spent the last three years of his life in a nursing home, and I experienced tremendous frustration when I would overnight a package containing a special dish that my father would enjoy. All the nursing home staff had to do was to microwave it for him. Instead, they would sign for it and let it sit and rot for several days at the main desk. And then, they would reprimand me for sending perishables.

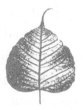

CHAPTER 21

BROUGHT TOGETHER BY BREAD AND CHEESE

People in farm villages did their best to help each other make it through the war years. Due to the shortage of food in the cities, the government required farmers who grew their own food to donate twenty percent of their crops to the local food bank. If they were caught not doing so, they received a hefty fine. My grandfather was not happy at all with that arrangement. He felt that farmers were working night and day just to feed their own families, and that the government could find other ways to feed the hungry population.

My shrewd grandfather always seemed to have a winning card up his sleeve. He knew the owner of the flour mill very well, so to avoid losing 20% of the wheat and to avoid the government inspectors, together they worked out a deal where for a small fee, my grandfather would be allowed to operate the mill a couple of nights a month. He would organize night trips to the mill with his daughters and other women on the farm. During the day, the women would transport the sacks of grain, by donkey or on their heads, to my grandfather's house. At night, they would re-load the heavy sacks onto their heads and quietly walk to the mill. While the mill was in operation, several people would hold watch posts to make sure no one would sneak up on them. Once they finished, the women would reload the sacks of flour on their heads and quietly walk back to my grandfather's house. By then it would be dawn, so they would load their sacks on the donkeys and head back home.

Bread was the main staple at every meal, accompanied by sautéed vegetables, cheese, zucchini omelet, or polenta, so it was crucial that every household had flour in the pantry at all times. Neighboring families would organize bread-making days so that they only needed to use one wood-burning brick oven at a time. Sometimes they would pool the flour and divvy up the bread once it was baked. Or they would bring their own prepared dough for baking along with other loaves.

They made the bread by mixing flour, water, and yeast in an oval wooden container made by hollowing out a tree trunk that was sanded and smoothed inside and out. It was large enough for two people to knead dough simultaneously. They probably used at least twenty to thirty pounds of flour for each batch. Once kneaded, the women allowed the dough to rise. Finally, they made the large, round loaves and left them to rise again. Once ready, they would slide the loaves into the wood-burning brick oven one at a time using a peel (a flat wooden shovel) with a long handle. It required a quick forward and backward jerking motion to release the loaf in the right place.

Particularly during the cold winter months, bread-making time gave the elders who suffered from arthritis an opportunity to enjoy a little relief. When the bread was fully baked, my grandmother would lie down on the bed on her stomach under a blanket. Her family members would then cover her, neck to toes with the hot loaves of bread as they came out of the oven. She would remain in that position for as long as she could tolerate the heat.

Cheese-making was also a communal effort. Participating families would contribute the milk they were able to get from their cows, goats, and sheep so that they had enough to make one big round of cheese. One of the families would take the round home to age on a wood rack hanging from the ceiling. Even though the ratio of three types of milk varied from batch to batch, the flavor of the cheese was always delicious.

CHAPTER 22

HOME FROM THE WAR

My father tried to sound hopeful and optimistic when he wrote to my mother during the war, "I hope you are taking good care of yourself and the baby. Don't worry about me. I am fine. The war will be over soon and I'll be home before you know it."

My mother had been worried sick since my father left, but she had become inconsolable with the loss of her brother Nicola. Numerous demanding chores on the farm kept her busy, but the fear of losing her husband in the war was forever present in her mind. She was dealt a further blow when she learned that my father had been captured and sent to a prisoner of war camp, first under the British and later under the Americans. There was probably not one family in the farm community who did not have a loved one away in the war, so luckily there was never a shortage of someone to talk to who could understand how she felt. It was this support that allowed everyone to survive the separation, the worry, and the fear during those years.

Because of the war, my oldest brother, Biagio, spent his first six years of life admiring my father only through a few pictures. He became very accustomed to having my mother all to himself. It became part of his mindset and he was contented with things the way they were.

When my father finally came home in 1946, Biagio was happy to meet him and was polite to him throughout the day. However, when it was bedtime on my father's first day home, Biagio went to my mother and asked her, "When is that man going to go home?"

She replied, "Biagio, honey, he is your father. He just got home, safe and sound. Hopefully, he'll never have to leave again."

"He's not my father," Biagio said as he ran to the nightstand. "This is daddy," he said as he ran back to my mother, holding one of the pictures she had received from my father during his years away.

My mother responded, "It's the same person!"

It took my brother some time to adjust to his new life with my father back home and having to share my mother with him. He resented my father for invading the cozy world he had relished his whole life with my mother and the extended family. He had been my mother's center of attention and now that was sadly over.

As we all know, soldiers who survive wars bring home deep emotional wounds and my father was no exception. Pampering my six-year-old brother was not acceptable behavior for a hardened soldier, and certainly not the way to raise him into a real man. After the initial homecoming festivities, it was back to work, work, work — only now, Biagio did not get to cling to my mother's apron strings. He had to follow my father's footsteps and grow up to be a man.

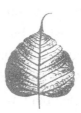

CHAPTER 23

THE WARM-UP ACT

In November 1946, my sister Maria was born and became one of millions forever to be known as "baby boomers." Fourteen months later, in February of 1948, my brother Nicola joined the family. Like every other couple separated by the years of war, my parents were busy making up for lost time.

The one-room house where they had settled right after they married was shrinking by the day, so building a new house became their main priority. Although resources were limited, the new place was going to have two large rooms with a storage attic, a chicken coop, a pigsty, a cage for rabbits, and a barn for wood and hay. They would build the new structure just 100 meters from the old place. Shortly after Nicola was born in February of 1948, construction started. New projects, new babies, and looking forward to a brighter future helped everyone leave the horrors of the war behind.

It was a huge undertaking to build a house without any efficient means to transport materials. Just to build a 400-square-foot, ground-level structure took a tremendous amount of preparation and careful coordination. Mules and donkeys hauled large stones, logs, and sacks of sand to the building site. Wheelbarrows and hand tools were the only non-breathing implements they used.

Women and children were, of course, part of the process. They gathered stones for the walls and carried them from the river to the construction site in baskets on their heads.

Once the workers had the foundation in place, they built the walls out of those precious hand-gathered stones and cemented them with mortar. They covered the outer surface with limestone and the interior with plaster. To get the limestone into a spreadable consistency, first they dug a big hole in the ground and then filled it with limestone and water carried from the creek. This created a chemical reaction that caused the limestone to melt into a hot paste. To keep it from hardening overnight, they covered it with dirt and leaves.

With two young children barely fourteen months apart, my mother had more than her share of responsibilities. Just to keep a fresh supply of clean diapers was a huge undertaking without a washing machine or running water. In those days, mothers kept newborns wrapped in fabric bands from the chest down like a log. They believed that it kept the baby's legs growing straight. It also made it easier to handle them and carry them safely in wicker bassinets.

In the early spring of 1950, my mother discovered that she was pregnant with her fourth child—me. I chose the last day of the year to join this chaotic world. I was the warm-up act for welcoming the New Year, born on December 31 at approximately 10:00 p.m. A few days later, my father went to city hall and reported the birth of his fourth child, Carmina. He recorded the time of birth to be January 1, 1951, shortly after midnight. He would later tell me that recording my birth on the first of January made it easier to calculate my age, and that to him, it just sounded better.

Progress on the new house was not moving as quickly as planned. My parents' dream was to complete the structure before my baptismal party. In the Catholic tradition, it is important to baptize children within the first three months of life to protect the soul of the newborn in case of death. Unbaptized innocent souls are believed to go to limbo rather than straight to Heaven. My little soul had to wait more than five months to be baptized until the new house was finished.

One day in late spring before construction was complete, my brother Nicola and my sister Maria were outside playing with our cousins, Maria and Pasqualina. The children were chasing each other around when my brother Nicola fell into the limestone pit. Luckily, the adults never lost sight of the children so my Aunt Teodora immediately jumped into action to pull him out. She carried him to the nearest water pond to wash him off. The limestone mixture was not at its hottest point, so fortunately he was not seriously hurt.

This incident ended well, but it raised some serious concerns about why Nicola would sometimes miss his step as though he could not see clearly where he was going. My parents promptly arranged for him to see a doctor. The diagnosis was not alarming. The doctor told them that Nicola had slightly blurry vision and that he might need glasses as he got older. This set their minds at ease and life returned to its normal rhythm.

By mid-June 1951, the new house was nearly finished. My parents scheduled my baptism party before completing the partition that would separate the two rooms; they wanted to have plenty of space for a nice, long table—and be able to dance and eat to their hearts' content.

My parents chose Giuseppe Sarubi, a cousin on my father's side, and his fiancée, Carmela, to be my godparents. They were madly in love with each other, but a tumultuous Shakespearian drama was evolving around them. As it happened, Giuseppe's sister and Carmela's brother were also dating. However, that relationship did not last. This unfortunate outcome infuriated my great aunt Rosina, Giuseppe's mother. As revenge, she demanded that Giuseppe break up with Carmela.

"If my daughter is not good enough for their son, then their daughter is not good enough for my son," Rosina would tell everyone. The would-be mothers-in-law of both couples had fierce words to say about each other's children. This discord put a damper on my mother's plans for my baptism. Giuseppe's mother asked my mother to select another couple to be my godparents, but my mother refused, insisting, "I don't care whether Carmela and Giuseppe get married or not, I want them to be my daughter's godparents." Giuseppe's mother reluctantly agreed.

CHAPTER 24

BRIGHT STARS, FULL MOON

I was baptized in mid-June 1951. After the church ceremony, everyone proceeded to the newly built house for a meal that lasted all day. My parents had slaughtered goats, sheep, rabbits, and chickens. They made pasta, bread, and cookies, and served their homemade wine. And of course, they had bought lots of Jordan almonds as party favors for all the guests. Dancing was always an important part of every party. There was never a shortage of accordion players to provide wonderful music for the *tarantellas* and other favorite local dances.

Dramatic love stories with lots of twists and turns have always captured attention, particularly in small farm communities where people don't have other types of entertainment. People in our community were no different. They were more than eager to speculate on the most recent gossip involving the relationship between Giuseppe and Carmela; some even went so far as to write songs predicting how the saga would end.

My godparents had not seen each other in several months, so the gossipmongers were all stirred up about the couple's reunion at my baptism. As the two of them stood together in church, all dressed up and holding me in my lacy baptismal gown, it became clear that the bickering between the two families had not destroyed their love. The rest of their day together was an excruciating ballet of soft gestures and warm glances, while trying not to attract the attention of Aunt Rosina or the gossipmongers. However, their first dance together was a prelude for long, secret embraces later on in the moonlight behind the haystacks.

None of the guests returned to their homes that night. Most of the women slept indoors on cornhusk mattresses either in the new house or the old one, while the men slept outside under the stars. No one in the family is sure where the lovebirds spent that night; somewhere in the galaxy of the heart, no doubt.

The peace did not last, however. Shortly after the last revelers had turned in for the night, the guard dogs began to bark continuously. People who were sober enough to hear them dismissed the barking as a reaction to the full moon. It was a beautiful warm night and some of the farm animals had been left in their outer pens. The dogs continued to bark frantically.

Suddenly the people sleeping in the old house heard loud screeching. They ran outside with their guns, firing warning shots. That was enough to scare off a pack of wolves that had probably been attracted to the house by all the cooking that day. But the shots fired were too late; the wolves had had enough time to kill about ten of the sheep and injure many more. The party-goers spent the rest of the night tending to the injured sheep. The next day, however, in the daylight, they determined the wounded sheep were not going to survive and that it would be best to discard all the meat, fearing possible diseases from the wolves.

I don't know how long the renewed relationship between my godparents went on, but it lasted long enough to make Giuseppe's mother spit fire when she found his bed full of garden squashes instead of his body after he snuck out of the house in the night to see his beloved Carmela. Realizing that she could not win this war alone, she mobilized a team of spies to help. Sooner or later she got her way, luckily without a Shakespearian ending. For the sake of family harmony, all four of the young lovers moved on and married other people. We will never know how happy they were. Without the combination of custom and family pride, things might have turned out differently.

I was only five and a half months old when the baptismal party took place, but I think I was left with an imprint of that very dramatic day. Maybe it is the reason why I've had a lifelong passion for great parties with unusual drama! And, while I doubt that sprinkling holy water on my forehead had any direct impact on my life, at least it created the circumstances surrounding an event that would long remind the Cantisani family of the wild nature of man and beast alike. Innocent though I was of all that went on that day, the telling of it has always featured my name, just as if the whole thing had somehow been my own doing. My mother always said that the day of my baptism was the basis of my tumultuous personality—extraordinarily fun or dangerously explosive— never anything in the middle.

Sometimes when I upset my mother, she would remind me of that fateful day. "It was a glorious summer day in June," she would say. She would go on to remind me that friends and family members came from near and far to partake in the festivities. The church ceremony was extra-special. The banquet was luscious and abundant. Everyone said how pretty you were. The accordion players never stopped playing, and people couldn't stop dancing. The stars were bright and the full moon was brilliant. Your lovesick godparents mended their hearts. But a hungry pack of wolves managed to put a bloody, sinister twist to what had been a most beautiful and memorable day.

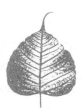

CHAPTER 25

THE BOMBSHELL DROPS

By the fall of 1951, my parents found themselves talking more and more about my brother Nicola's eyesight. They were confused about the way he sometimes zipped around the farm as though he could see perfectly, then other times depended on my older sister Maria to help him find things he had dropped on the ground. They decided to take him to an eye specialist in Potenza, the capital of the Basilicata region. It was an all-day journey and I got to go along because I was still nursing.

The doctor examined my brother and then, to my mother's surprise, asked to examine me. "What for?" my mother replied, "Her eyes are as bright as they can be and she focuses on everything perfectly. Last night she was pointing at the full moon."

"Go ahead, let the doctor see her," my father said. "That way we can rest assured." So my mother agreed to the doctor's request. He examined and re-examined both Nicola and me to make certain he was really seeing what he was seeing. His behavior concerned my parents right away, but as was common in Italy, doctors do not converse with their patients during the examination.

Finally he put down his equipment and pushed back his chair. My mother picked me up from the examination table and sat me on her lap. My father was standing next to Nicola, restless with anticipation.

The doctor dropped the bombshell.

"Both your children suffer from a degenerative eye disease called Retinitis Pigmentosa. It is a condition passed on by a recessive gene to some of the offspring when both parents carry it. It is very rare, however, to find the manifestation of this gene in offspring of both genders. Unfortunately there is no cure for this disease."

A long pause followed. My parents looked at him as if he were speaking in a foreign language. The doctor realized that my parents had not been able to process anything he had just said, except maybe that there was no cure. Their demeanor broke his heart. He needed to repeat everything he had just said, only this time slowly, in a simplified manner, and with compassion.

"Your children are not completely blind," he said, "They just have limited vision for now."

"What do you mean, limited vision?" asked my father.

"It means that they can see what's around them, but not see very far. For example, the details that we see at a distance of 20 feet, they will see only if they are much closer, perhaps two to three feet. They can see contrast, so if they drop something and it is a different color than the floor, they can see it, but if it blends in they might not see it."

My father sighed in disbelief. My mother was totally confused.

"I know that it's a difficult thing to hear, but don't despair," the doctor continued. "There are schools for blind children. They can get an education and become successful like everybody else."

"You mean there's no operation that can be done?" asked my father.

"No, not at the moment, but maybe in the future there will be. Medical science is constantly improving."

The doctor decided that it was better to omit the rest of the information regarding the disease for now. Eventually he would have to tell my parents that as their children grew older, they would eventually lose whatever functional vision they had.

Everything my parents had known about life up to that moment was irreparably changed. They were hearing words they had never heard before and they could not comprehend their meaning. How could they suddenly have two blind children who would not be able to go to school with regular kids and learn to read and write? How could these children live and work on a farm where deadly accidents were always just one moment of distraction away? What had they done wrong to deserve this?

My mother's knees buckled. She staggered when she tried to take a step. Everything in front of her eyes looked dark and twisted. She thought about me growing old without a husband or a family because no man would want to marry a blind woman unable to take care of her children and her household. And Nicola? How could he work and support a family?

The feeling of guilt and despair nearly choked her. She could hardly breathe. I must have done something seriously wrong in my life and God is punishing me for it now, she thought, but what? The last time she had gone to confession she had confided to the priest about her worries over Nicola's blurry vision. The priest had told her to pray more. Maybe she hadn't prayed enough and now God was punishing her.

My father, a much less religious person than my mother, decided that the specialist was a quack and that he didn't know what he was talking about. My father believed that the first doctor had given the correct diagnosis: Nicola's vision was a little blurry and he might need glasses. As for me, my eyes just looked too perfect to have anything wrong with them.

This visit to the eye specialist initiated a life-long battle between my parents. As my oldest brother Biagio often put it in later years, "World War II was over in 1945, but our family war began in 1951. Your blindness was the beginning of a standoff that just kept them at odds. Our father's stubborn nature and inability to accept reality kept him in turmoil for the rest of his life and our mother suffered profound sadness and guilt for nearly all of hers. They started fighting about which solutions would give you a better future and then their arguments flowed over into everything."

When we were finally back at the farm, the news traveled quickly through our extended family. Everyone seemed to take my father's view: the doctor in Potenza must be a quack. Nicola didn't look blind, and I was too much of a happy, bouncy toddler with beautiful brown eyes to lend credibility to the quack's diagnosis. My mother, desperate to feel better about the situation, wholeheartedly welcomed the extra fuel for denial.

Through the winter months of 1951 and 1952, Nicola and I stayed indoors, out of danger. My parents were content avoiding the truth. Maria acted as my full-time babysitter and Biagio kept Nicola happy with his passion for building toy-size farm equipment. They would collect pieces of wood and raid my father's box of brand-new nails. When my father discovered that, he was not happy. He told Nicola to collect used nails from old lumber that had been discarded.

My brother obeyed, and with someone's help he would straighten old nails with a hammer. One day in the spring of 1952, while trying to build a miniature plow, Nicola dropped a nail on the ground. The nail was small and didn't create enough of a contrast on the ground for him to find it. He became frustrated and called out for Maria to help. My mother was watching. The truth suddenly hit her like the proverbial ton of bricks. At last she understood that the eye specialist in Potenza was right. My father was wrong and so was everyone else who had sided with him. For sure Nicola was blind.

Together with Aunt Teodora, my mother started testing my brother's eye sight. They would drop things on the floor and watch him try to retrieve them. My brother's performance was that of a little boy with limited vision. Sometimes he would find the items and sometimes he wouldn't, even if they were very close to him. My mother and my aunt looked at each other with tears in their eyes, saying over and over, "Oh my dear Jesus, what are we going to do?"

The truth was obvious, and the relentless quest for a cure began. The entire farm community mobilized into action. Aunts, uncles, first cousins, second cousins, cousins once, twice, three times removed, grandparents, great aunts and uncles, godparents, and their extended families and friends—all looked for doctors, eye specialists, even palm-readers, psychics, or priests who could wash our eyes with holy water or invoke special Latin prayers asking God to grant us a miracle.

My Aunt Teodora, my father's sister, her husband, Egidio, and their three children, Maria, Lina, and Nicola, were always present and involved in every decision my parents made because we functioned together as one family. In our home, the rules were clear: with the help of Teodora's family, my older brother Biagio, twelve, and my sister Maria, six, were now responsible for most of the farm chores while my parents took Nicola and me all over Southern Italy looking for a cure. Too young to understand what this was doing to my family, I loved these excursions to no end. The passion for travel was in my blood and I looked forward to every trip, long or short, with excitement.

Before each journey, Maria would diligently help my mother get us ready. She would feed me spoonful after spoonful of homemade chicken broth with *pastina* (small, star-shaped pasta or other small pasta), followed by bite after bite of homemade bread dunked in a sunny-side-up egg gathered from the chicken coop that morning. Sunny-side-up eggs were everyone's favorite, but eggs were not plentiful; therefore, they were usually only prepared for children with fussy eating habits or for unexpected guests.

Biagio would help my father get the donkey ready: saddle him up and secure a wicker basket on either side of the saddle. Once Nicola and I were loaded into the baskets and the weight was well balanced, the journey would begin. Biagio, Maria, and Aunt Teodora would tell us to be careful and to go slowly, and then they would stand in front of the house sadly waving goodbye until they lost sight of us.

At the start of each trip, everyone hoped and prayed that this was going to be the time we would return home with a treatment or a cure. The remedies suggested by psychics and other charlatans kept everyone temporarily hopeful. One suggested treatment included putting drops of breast milk from nursing women into our eyes. Catholic priests, of course, were never bashful to promise my mother they would say special prayers in Latin in return for a donation. Our house was full of church artifacts representing saints, Jesus figurines in all sizes and shapes and, of course, enough Holy Marys and angels to put the high Heavens to shame.

My parents' lack of exposure and literacy was not what created the impenetrable wall of ignorance around them. They were simply reacting like loving parents to an avalanche of life-altering, incorrect information. Once they had exhausted all of the leads for possible cures, my mother insisted on returning to the eye specialist in Potenza. My mother was a woman with unusual intuition and resolve. She was going to find out from this eye specialist what kind of future was possible for her blind children, and she was not going to leave his office until she received all the information she wanted.

The specialist told my parents that blind children could receive an education in residential schools for the blind. The nearest such school was in Naples, an entire day's travel from where we lived. Hearing this news that we could get an education and become self-sufficient, lifted a huge weight off my parents' shoulders, but almost immediately a new weight saddled their emotions: it meant that once we reached school age, they would have to put us in this school permanently until we graduated from high school or a trade school at the age of 18.

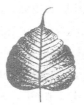

CHAPTER 26

WITNESS TO PAIN

Amid the turmoil of this rollercoaster my parents were riding, my mother discovered she was pregnant again! And now the sky really did fall on her. Her thoughts started spinning out of control. She had run out of people to see and places to go hoping for a solution to what she saw as a horrible disgrace from God. She didn't need priests to tell her it was sacrilege to even think of terminating her pregnancy. She didn't need doctors to tell her they were not going to help her abort the fetus. And she certainly did not need the entire farm community pitying her, the poor woman who kept giving birth to blind children.

My mother plunged into a deep depression. My father became taciturn and lost his temper easily. He snapped at Biagio and Maria when things didn't go exactly his way. He hadn't yet realized that snapping at blind children was not a mortal sin, so for the time being, Nicola and I were spared. My mother was too sad and too pregnant to be snapped at. The mood at home became bleak. Morning after morning we watched my mother sit by the fire, elbows on her knees, holding her face between her hands, her beautiful waist-length hair draped over her shoulders, crying inconsolably. The fear that she was going to give birth to another blind child completely destroyed her.

After a while, she would become angry. She would quickly braid her hair, pin it around the back of her head, and go about her chores, banging things around as hard as she could. When she went to the pond to do the wash, she would dunk each item in the icy water that came from melting snow on the higher peaks. She would slam it on the rock and rub it with a big cake of olive soap and then scrub the hell out of it angrily as she cried and prayed aloud to Jesus. By the time she was finished, her hands would be as red as though covered with blood.

We watched our mother weep every day, and there wasn't a thing we could do to comfort her. It is so true what they say: It's more painful to witness pain than to experience it. We would have done anything to help her. Meanwhile, her Catholic priest could have lifted her guilt at any time during her confessions. He could have told her that having blind children was not a punishment from God, that blindness has existed since the beginning of time, and that some blind people even became priests. If my mother had heard these words it would have helped her feel human again. But of course, it didn't happen.

Nevertheless, the normal cycle of life on the farm had to continue even in the face of the emotional chaos my mother suffered. Slowly but surely, we made it through the gloomy days preceding Easter. During the forty days of Lent only the children and the sick were allowed to eat an occasional small serving of meat. The families participated in prayer vigils, processions, the carrying of the cross, confessions, and masses one after another. Especially during the last week leading up to the resurrection of Jesus Christ.

On Palm Sunday, the Sunday before Easter, people symbolically made peace with each other by exchanging olive branches. Everyone who could was expected to go to confession and receive communion on Easter Sunday. I was too young for any of these things, except eating the delicious Easter bread that my mother had made one or two days before. We were not allowed to eat any of the bread until Easter morning, well after the resurrection of Christ.

The youngest children in the family always received a loaf of Easter bread in the shape of a doll. A hard-boiled egg was placed in the center of the head where you could draw a face. I didn't like taking bites of the doll and watching it disappear piece by piece, so I chose to eat my Easter bread from the regular loaf.

The hustle and bustle of springtime farm activities—making cheese, washing and shearing the sheep, and planting new crops—made summer come around very quickly. For our family, that was a good thing. My mother was simply too busy and distracted to think about anything but the present moment. The numerous summer harvests kept us in the company of so many people all the time that my mother's demeanor seemed once again happy and healthy. She looked forward to having the new baby and she hoped that with the help and good grace of God, he or she would be healthy and sighted.

Harvest time involved nonstop work for the adults and older children, but for the younger ones, it meant just lots and lots of playtime. We would stop playing only when we were called to eat. I remember hearing the loud, long yodel calls from the women who brought the homemade cooked meal to the field in the early afternoon. We would run to the tree-shaded area where my mother and the other women were lowering the big linen-wrapped wicker baskets from their heads to the ground. They had to repeatedly encourage the workers to come and eat, calling, "Come on, come on, it's time to eat. You have worked enough for now!"

It was considered impolite to stop working as soon as the food arrived: one was to stand on ceremony and wait to be encouraged to partake in the meal. As the women unwrapped the wicker baskets, the wonderful aroma of food permeated the air. First, we ate the homemade gnocchi or cavatelli coated with a rabbit stew sauce and sprinkled with homemade cheese. Then, fried peppers with nuggets of homemade sausage, homemade bread, and a salad of just-picked tomatoes and cucumbers. Work for the adults and playtime for the children would resume only after a long rest. That was mandatory. They believed it was unhealthy to work immediately after a meal.

CHAPTER 27

FIRST EXPOSURE TO CRUELTY

One late afternoon, toward the end of the corn harvest, I was playing with a group of children around the pond-like area where my mother usually did the wash. Some older boy noticed a black cat drinking the water. "Let's drown the cat," he said. "Black cats bring bad luck."

The boys all grabbed long sticks and started pushing the cat under the water. The cat swam to the other side of the pond and frantically try to climb out, gasping for air and hissing at the boys when he could. But before he could get away the boys would run to catch him and quickly push him down again until the cat was exhausted and full of water. It was happening very quickly and I couldn't really see what was happening, but I wanted the cat to get away. I had a sick feeling in my stomach. I was revolted and repulsed by the entire thing. I knew deep inside, that something really bad was going to happen to the cat.

The cat finally drowned. The boys then left laughing as though they had just heard a funny story. I on the other hand, remained on the scene with deep sadness, leaning against the tall tree that arched over the pond, wishing that the cat had gotten away safely. I could see the rippling water sparkling like a thousand little mirrors in the low afternoon sun.

As I moved my gaze toward the shady part of the pond where I could see things more clearly, I spotted the dead cat floating. Until that moment I had never been able to get a good look at a cat because they were not allowed in the house. Outdoors they always moved much too quickly for me to really see them. Now, here was my chance. First I saw his long tail, slightly curved, then his hindquarters, then his bloated belly, then his front quarters, and finally his droopy head. I was alone for a few minutes before anyone came. I felt sick as I stared and stared at the dead cat. I wanted him not to be dead.

Soon I heard my father coming towards the pond, talking with someone. He noticed me standing next to the tree. "Carmelina, what are you doing there by yourself?"

"Nothing ..."

"There's a dead cat floating in the water; do you know what happened?" asked my father.

"The boys pushed him under the water with long sticks," I said, with tears in my eyes. "Why did they do that?"

"Because they are stupid, Carmelina!" my father said. "But, don't worry my little one, there are other cats on the farm."

My father went for a rake, pulled the cat from the water and away he trudged. I have never been able to wipe that awful image from my memory. I wish I hadn't spotted the cat at all. I continue trying to find some logical explanation as to why people do the things they do. It was my first exposure to cruelty.

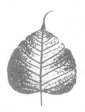

CHAPTER 28

PIETRO COMES SCREAMING INTO THE WORLD

On the morning of September 27, 1954, right in the middle of winemaking season, before my mother even had a chance to go out and start the day, her water broke. Immediately children of responsible age ran to the nearest dwellings to deliver the news. In turn, children from these dwellings would fan out to more distant homes spreading the word further.

As with every birth, plans for the delivery had been made far in advance. In less than an hour, women began arriving to help my mother with the labor. Aunt Teodora, who lived only a couple of hundred yards away, was there from the first holler. Within a short time our house was full of women to attend to my mother's every need.

Men and children were not allowed inside. I remember spending a long time playing with my siblings, my cousins, and other children just below the house in the flat, round area used in the summertime for threshing wheat. At one point I climbed the little hill and walked toward the house. It must have been late afternoon. I could tell from the familiar elongated shadows on the house. I heard my father rushing out the door. He told me to go back to playing and he hurried in the direction of the donkey's stall. Soon he emerged on the donkey trotting down the hill as fast as the donkey would go.

Years later I would learn my father had been rushing to town to find a professional midwife because my mother was having life-threatening labor complications. The baby was breach and could not be delivered normally. My mother appeared to be near death. Aunt Teodora declared that a mother of five could not be allowed to die so she took matters into her own hands. She pulled the baby out.

Sadly, the umbilical cord was wrapped around the baby's neck and she was dead. The women did their very best as always, but they were not prepared to resolve such serious complications. The lifeless body was handed to one of the aunts who pronounced her name to be Mattia and performed baptism rights for the unfortunate child.

Much to everyone's surprise a second baby was waiting to be delivered. The second baby, my brother Pietro, came screaming into the world, much to everyone's relief.

Meanwhile, having reached the town, my father was lucky to find a professional midwife. But the woman was old and afraid to ride on a donkey. She, however, was not shy about holding onto the donkey's tail for extra support as she and my father undertook the two hour walk to reach our house. By the time my father and midwife appeared, the babies had already made their arrival. When the midwife joined my mother in the bedroom, my mother was experiencing such excruciating abdominal pain that she was unable to speak. The midwife grabbed my mother's belly with both hands and began using a repeated sweeping motion from my mother's chest down. This procedure caused my mother to scream as she had never screamed before; but after a while she began to feel some relief.

As with all family lore, the details change with the viewpoint of the storyteller, but the one constant in it all is that Aunt Teodora saved my mother's life during the birth of the twins. The tragedy of losing baby Mattia was offset in everyone's minds because, unlike Pietro and his siblings, she would not have to live with blindness.

My mother had known all along, based on what doctors had told her, that Pietro would be born blind. Once she had given birth to one child suffering from Retinitis Pigmentosa, all future children would have the same eye disease. To my mother, Pietro's blindness was a tragedy in itself.

For weeks, women from both sides of our extended family hovered like bees around my mother, taking care of each and every one of her needs, which is a rare luxury that women got to enjoy only after giving birth. Her only responsibilities were to eat, rest, and breastfeed her newborn.

When she finally regained her strength and was able to resume her activities, her younger children, whom had been staying with relatives, were allowed to return home. During this time I got to stay with my famous great aunt Rosina (my godfather Giuseppe's mother). When it was time to return home I asked her to put me in a wicker basket and carry me on her head, because I wanted to remember what it was like to be carried in a wicker basinet. Of course she agreed because she liked to spoil me. With each step my great aunt Rosina took, I could feel the top of her head poking through the basket.

I had conflicted feelings about returning home. I had always liked being the youngest in the family and was not ready to share my mother's attention with a little brother. At the same time, I liked the idea of having a younger sibling I could boss around the way my older siblings tried to boss me around. When my mother saw Rosina arriving with me on her head, she yelled, "What are you doing? She's too heavy. Put her down, you are going to hurt your neck!"

"Oh, nonsense," my great aunt Rosina replied, "she doesn't even weigh as much as a barrel of water." She lifted the basket from her head and put it on the ground. I climbed out of the basket and ran to my mother.

"You got big!" she said to me. "Did Aunt Rosina feed you ten times a day?" Happy as I had been with my great aunt's family, I was ecstatic to see my mother, and it was wonderful to be home. She wasn't holding the baby so she scooped me into her lap and kissed me on both cheeks. My great aunt Rosina quickly went into the bedroom to see the baby, then immediately found chores she could do around our house for my mother.

The earliest memory I have of my little brother is lying next to him on my parents' bed while my mother was changing him. She told me I was not allowed to touch his face. I could touch his hand and his arm, but that was all!

At one point, she left the room to get something from the kitchen and that's when curiosity got the best of me. His hands were shaped into fists, small and smooth, not scuffed up like everyone else's hands from working on the farm. I worked my way up his tiny arm, his neck, his miniature ears, and finally his fuzzy head. I felt around the top of his head and was intrigued to discover a soft spot. I wondered what would happen if I pushed in a little bit on the soft spot. I did push in a little bit and the soft spot went in slightly.

At that moment, my mother returned to the bedroom and chased me away with a slap on my buttocks, screaming, "You can ruin his brain by doing that! I told you not to touch him! Why are you so disobedient?" To this day, I tease my younger brother about being the way he is because I squished his brain out of place when he was a tiny baby.

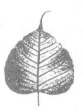

CHAPTER 29

OF SNOW AND BUTTER

The euphoria that accompanies a new arrival in the family kept everyone distracted, at least for a while. However, slowly but surely life regained its normal rhythm. In October of 1955, I started seeing my little brother Pietro dressed in a long, navy blue robe with a large, round, white collar and a white, rope-like belt, after he was no longer wearing his wraps. He looked like a miniature priest. I was told this was a replica of the robe worn by Saint Anthony. In her prayers, my mother had promised Saint Anthony that she would dress my little brother in the saint's robe for one year as a sign of devotion, hoping that Saint Anthony would help Pietro get his sight. At least this kept my mother hoping for something instead of crying herself into total despair.

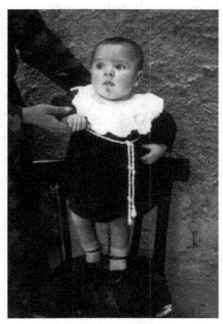

Pietro (Peter) in Saint Anthony robe.

It was also during this time that Nicola made his first long journey to the residential School for the Blind in Naples. My father and Biagio accompanied him. While they were gone, I remember sleeping in the big bed in my father's spot. My mother would ask me to blow out the oil lamp every night after reciting our bedtime prayers. We were not quite sure how long the trip would take, but our dog knew to the moment when they would be home. As soon as my father and Biagio began the one-hour climb from town, our dog sat in front of the house and howled. I think it was this that engendered in me a profound appreciation and love for dogs. What could be more impressive than the love and devotion of a dog for his master and the way it shows itself?

I don't know how things went for Nicola during his first months away from home, but for me Christmas seemed to roll around pretty quickly. From time to time my mother would sigh deeply and ask Jesus in a soft voice, "I wonder how that little boy is doing?"

I don't remember anything unusual about the holidays, but I have clear memories of the day Nicola set out for the journey back to school. He was sitting by the fireplace eating his breakfast, a large slice of homemade bread, probably with cheese and prosciutto on it. He was leaning forward, keeping his knees wide apart to make sure he didn't get any crumbs on his dress uniform—navy blue wool pants with suspenders and a crisp white shirt that my mother had ironed the day before with a charcoal iron. His shoes were covered with socks to keep dust or ashes off them. I stood behind him thinking how important he seemed now! He was going to school and wearing such impressive clothes.

It had snowed heavily the night before, and my father was trying to convince him to wait another day until the weather cleared. Six-year-old Nicola wouldn't hear of it. "If I arrive at school one day late, I'll never be able to catch up with the others!" So, dangerous as it was, my father readied the donkey and they set out for the long trip. As usual, my father boarded the donkey in Castelluccio Inferiore and they proceeded by bus and train to Naples.

I don't remember how many days it took for my father to return home, but it seemed like a very long time. It continued to snow to the point where there was nothing to do but to stay inside and pray we wouldn't die buried by the snow. When it finally stopped snowing, it took families days to carve their way out of their houses. We were isolated from the rest of the world for weeks and weeks.

My father had made it back from Naples only as far as the town of Castelluccio Inferiore. And there he waited until it stopped snowing and enough snow melted so that it was possible for him and the donkey to attempt the climb home. We had no way of knowing what might have happened to him; we worried and prayed every waking moment, hoping he would make it home safe and sound. We all knew the day had arrived when he decided it was safe enough to climb up the hills because the dog sat in front of the house and started howling for hours on end until he could see my father and the donkey in the distance. We were relieved and thankful he'd made it home. We had just lived through the big snowstorm of 1956, one of the biggest on record for Southern Italy.

The next morning, my father was standing outside in front of the house and saw something in the sky. He shouted urgently, "Come see, come see!" We all ran outside wondering what was going on. "There is an American helicopter dropping food aid," he said. We had never seen a helicopter before, so it was exciting for us. I couldn't actually see the helicopter, but I could hear it. I fell in love with Americans at that moment.

Apparently the American military base in Naples had organized the aid mission to drop food to the rural areas that had been isolated by this historic snowstorm. My father was as proud as he could be to have been a war prisoner under the Americans. "The Americans know how to do things! They don't sit around and wait for people to starve to death before deciding to organize a rescue mission," he said, adding, "I'm going to town to see how they are going to distribute the goods." Biagio went with him along with the donkey because they thought they were going to bring home lots of goodies.

We waited, bursting with excitement, jumping around at the prospect of eating new treats. Father and Biagio returned rather quickly. The wicker baskets hanging on both sides of the donkey saddle were not overflowing with packages and neither my father nor my brother looked particularly overjoyed.

As they came within hearing distance, I heard my father swear for the first time in my life. He went on and on in his rage. Apparently, the

Americans had, in good faith, dropped the food aid at the church, but the priests were giving out only one big can of butter and one big can of powdered milk per family. If you wanted more than that, you had to buy it from them. I began to wonder why my parents were so loyal to the church when the Catholic establishment and even the faith itself seemed more a source of disappointment than of grace.

It was a beautiful, bright morning the next day. I was outside playing in the fluffy white snow when my father called me inside, "Here, try this," he said. It was a slice of my mother's homemade bread with American butter on it and sprinkled with sugar. It was my first time tasting butter. I still can't forget the wonderful surprise my taste buds experienced that morning thanks to the Americans.

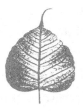

CHAPTER 30

BUTCHERING DAY

I enjoyed getting older. I was five now, and everyone was telling me that the following fall I would be going to go away to school like Nicola. I liked the sound of that and looked forward to learning new things and growing up smart. From then on I made sure I followed my mother everywhere she went so I could learn to be just like her. "You are a girl," she'd say. "You need to learn how to do everything around the house and on the farm, and go to school; otherwise, you won't find a husband when you grow up."

It made me a little sad to hear that because I was already five and had not learned how to do too many things yet. I would have to learn how to go to town by myself like she did, and that seemed so difficult. My mother always knew her way and never got lost. I was afraid I would never learn and one day I would get lost in the woods and be eaten by wolves.

As soon as the snow melted enough so that people could get around after the big snowstorm, it was time to slaughter the hog that every family had been fattening up for the past year. I had gone to the pigsty with my mother almost every day to feed the hog. I liked to watch him inhale the food we put in front of him. I was never allowed to touch him.

"He's dirty," my mother would say, "and you're small; he might bite you."

"He looks good, God bless him. He is going to bring abundance to the family, God willing," people would comment about each other's hogs.

It was cool and overcast the morning of the big event.

"Perfect weather. God must be on our side for a change. We have nothing to complain about, for once" my father claimed as he briskly continued to get his work area ready outside. My father was going to be slaughtering our hog himself. He was regarded as one of the best butchers in the area. His dexterity with a knife was greatly admired.

I stood by the doorway as everyone walked briskly in and out of the house getting coordinated so that once the pig was killed each task could be tackled immediately. Once everything was ready, everyone came inside except for my father and the other men who were in charge of slaughtering the pig. They went to the sty to get him.

I thought about the numerous times I had gone there with my mother to feed him and now that was coming to an end. I stood on my toes just behind the closed, bottom portion of the Dutch door. All of the activities were happening in front of the house and much of it was close enough for me to see. As soon as I saw the hog emerge and heard his grunting, all the blood in my body rushed to my legs. I nearly fainted. I grabbed the door to help me stay on my feet. I wanted to run to the pig, to help him escape and hide somewhere.

But almost immediately he was hoisted onto a bench, tied up securely and stabbed in the throat. I heard the most frightening, loud, screeching scream as the knife went in. I prayed and trembled as the screeching grew weaker and weaker. I was so sad. I wondered why I couldn't be happy and excited like the rest of the children and the grown-ups who were celebrating the death of this animal.

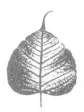

CHAPTER 31

OFF TO BOARDING SCHOOL

In the fall of 1956, at age five-and-a-half, it was time for me to leave home and go away to the boarding School for the Blind. Everyone in my family and beyond had been talking to me for months about all the wonderful things I was going to learn there and how much fun I was going to have. "When you come back, we won't recognize you! We won't even understand you. You will be speaking proper Italian. You will be a city girl. Your skin won't be so dark anymore from spending so much time outside. You'll get used to living with running water and electricity. Each room will be lighted with bright lights. The floors will be clean and shiny. You'll never be covered with smoke or ashes from these old fireplaces or burning unseasoned wood. At school, they can just push a button to turn on the heat. You'll be able to take a bath in a big tub where hot water comes out straight from a faucet. You'll be able to eat meat a least once a day."

I had so much to look forward to I could hardly wait to go to boarding school. I was sure that I was going to love it. As the day of the big trip approached, I became ecstatic. I could hardly sleep. The morning of the trip I woke up way before the wind-up alarm clock went off. I could not wait for my mother to help me get ready. She had sewn a brand-new dress and coat; and had knitted beautiful wool socks to go with my outfit. I also had new shoes, the kind you only wear in the city: smooth and shiny on top with smooth soles on the bottom. I had never worn anything like that before and I was in Heaven.

It was still dark outside when my father hoisted Nicola and me into the wicker baskets mounted on either side of the donkey saddle. We said goodbye to Maria, Biagio, and Aunt Teodora, and away we went. I don't remember saying goodbye to two-year-old Pietro. He was probably still sleeping. I remember hearing the comforting sounds of my parents' footsteps as they kept pace with the donkey going down the hill. I could hear the sounds of the donkey's hooves on the rocks and the rushing water as we passed little streams every now and then. The air smelled cool and fresh and the sun was still not up. Everything was calm except for my thoughts.

I don't remember being lifted out of the basket once we reached Castelluccio Inferiore, but I do remember the bus ride to the train station. As soon as the bus started moving, I started screaming, "Whoa, whoa!" as if slowing down a donkey or a horse. The bus was moving much too fast for me and I was really scared. My mother tried her best to calm me. She didn't want the other passengers to know I had never been on a bus before except when I was too young to remember.

Some nice ladies sitting in front of us reached back and tried to hand me some candy. I had to turn it down initially because it was impolite to accept something at first offering. I had to stand on ceremony. Luckily, they insisted many times and finally my mother gave in. "Go ahead. You can take it, but thank the nice ladies for being so kind."

They had partially removed the foil from what would be the most delicious thing I would ever taste in my life. As soon as I put it in my mouth and it started melting, I must have left the planet for a few seconds. When I finally came to, the candy called chocolate had already slid down my throat, leaving behind the most uncontrollable urge for more. I remember promising myself the very first thing I would do with my first paycheck as a grown-up: I would spend it all on CHOCOLATE. I would go to an isolated place and eat it all, non-stop. With my second paycheck I would buy more and perhaps share a little bit of it.

We got off the bus in Potenza to walk the rest of the way to the train station. The ground was smooth and hard. I could walk without stumbling on anything. My new shoes remained nice and clean, and so did my new outfit. The streets were lined on either side with tall houses. Some had big glass windows with beautiful things on display. My mother explained to me those were called stores, "… that's where people who have money can buy things."

All the sounds were new and different. My mother even let me feel a parked car. "This is how people get around in the city. They don't use donkeys like us." Now that I'd seen a car I had something else I wanted to buy with my first paycheck, even though my parents told me that I could not see well enough to drive. When I grew up, I was not going to be blind anymore anyway, so I could drive a car. And besides, I would buy a small one without a roof so that I could see everything around me. I wished that my parents would move to the city. I never wanted to go back to the farm again.

I soon began daydreaming about my exciting and happy future in the city. No more mud or puddles to step into and get all dirty. No more rocks and bushes to walk through and no more cow pies to worry about falling into. And for sure, no more smoky smell from the fireplace. My mind was filled with new thoughts that went on and on in every direction, so much so I don't remember the rest of the trip.

When we finally arrived in Naples it was dark again. I remember that my left arm was stretching way up in the air to hold my father's hand. In my right hand I was carrying my plastic school bag with a package of store-bought cookies. I'd never eaten store-bought cookies before, and I could not wait to have some. The streets were wet from the rain, but there was no mud or puddles. Occasionally on either side of the street, a pole with a light on top of it shone much brighter than our oil lamp at the farm.

"We are almost there. It's going to be nice and warm inside," my father said. We soon approached a gate on the right. The two lampposts on either side really made it stand out. We walked through the gate and immediately to the left was a tiny house. Someone opened a window and my father announced our name. Then he turned to me and said, "That's where the gatekeeper lives." The gatekeeper pushed a button and said into the intercom, "The Cantisanis are here." Then he turned toward us and said to go right ahead.

We walked along a paved path with trees on both sides. The path widened into a large round area. Facing us was a four-story building. The school was exactly as Nicola described, built like a monastery. We proceeded under a tall archway that led us into an interior courtyard. On the ground level all along the left side the doors of the chapel stood with their stained-glass windows; on the right, carports with marble staircases led in different directions. Straight ahead were two big double doors. The one on the left opened as we approached. A woman dressed in a black uniform with a white collar greeted us.

We entered a large, square room with a round table in the center and chairs along each wall. "This is the visiting room," my father said, "where the families visit with their children." As he said that, he lifted me onto the table. I noticed how bright everything looked. I could see around the room as though it was daylight, but it was nighttime.

"Can you see the light?" my father asked. "See how nice and bright it is?" The light came from a round tube in the ceiling making everything look just like it did in the sunlight. A strange, unfamiliar feeling came over me. I asked myself, Why do the parents have to come here to talk with their children? Don't they sleep with them?

The lady who had let us in sat down at a desk in the corner to write something. Shortly thereafter, a second woman came into the room through a different door. She was wearing the same black uniform with a white collar. She walked over to me and said, "You must be Carmelina, Nicola Cantisani's sister! You are so pretty! Who made this beautiful dress for you?"

"My mother," I replied in a shy voice, but I was happy to hear that someone from the city liked my dress. It must be really beautiful.

"Would you like to come play with the other children?" she asked.

Almost simultaneously, my mother reached over to kiss me and said, "Be a good girl for the teacher and we'll come visit you soon."

My father added, "If you're a good girl, we'll bring you chocolates, like the one you ate this morning on the bus, remember? You'd like that, wouldn't you?"

As the teacher tried to pick me up and carry me away, my world as I knew it ended.

The tube of light on the ceiling lost its shape as my eyes overflowed with a long stream of tears. As my body filled with fear and despair I became an unapproachable ball of fire. I kicked, punched, screamed, scratched, bit. Everything went flying off the table and landed in different directions. I have no memory of what followed for the rest of the evening.

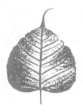

CHAPTER 32

FIRST DAY AT SCHOOL

My next memory is of waking up in a long, rectangular room with a row of single beds on either side. At the end of each row of beds stood a white tent surrounding a bed where the proctor slept. My bed was on the outer wall next to the balconies. Standing next to my bed was a child about my sister's age.

"I'm going to help you get dressed," she said.

"Where's my mommy?" I asked.

"She'll come later. Put your arms up so I can slip off your nightgown." She removed my nightgown and helped me put on first an undershirt, then a slip, then a dark wool dress, and then a long-sleeved, button-down, blue-and-white-checkered, cotton knee-length uniform smock. Beige ankle socks and black Mary Jane shoes completed the outfit that every female student in the school wore. The boys wore dark blue smocks; and all the staff wore black smocks with a white collar.

My helper took me to the bathroom and assisted me in using the toilet, something only my mother had done before. We then walked over to a long sink with a row of faucets where I washed my hands and face. All these things were new and different, but all I wanted was to be back on the farm. She combed my hair, and according to the rules, I was ready for the day.

At 7:15 sharp, an adult from under the tent shouted, "It's time to get in line, girls!"

Every child took a designated spot in a line of twos, holding hands, the shortest children in the front, graduating to the tallest in the back. Once we were all in our proper spots, the proctor inspected each of us to ensure we were properly dressed and groomed. If just one child didn't pass muster, the group could not proceed until the problem was corrected. She warned us not to utter a sound once we left the room. We all moved forward, looking exactly the same, just like little prisoners.

Other groups of older children already waited in formation on the large landing, all set to go downstairs. Two of those groups were boys who had come down from the upper floor; and I knew that among them would be my brother Nicola. I could feel his presence. As soon as our group was given the go-ahead, we walked down three flights of marble stairs two-by-two, holding hands. The proctor stayed at the front of the line, giving orders as necessary. Sounds echoed in this large stairwell, and you could hear the footsteps of all the children from the ground floor all the way to the top floor.

Immediately to the right of the last set of stairs were the double doors that opened to the dining rooms. We were headed for the chapel before breakfast, so we kept on going straight. We walked through another set of dark double doors that led us to the visiting room. My heart started pounding as we walked through that room where I had last seen my parents. I could smell the cigarette smoke coming from the adjacent office, where Miss Antonacci, the school director, sat at her desk. As my group entered the room, everyone shouted in unison: "Good morning Madam Director!" In a serious tone she replied, "Good morning, children."

The sunlight from the bay window at the end of the room illuminated the faces of a man and a woman standing in a corner to my left. They seemed to be my parents. Were they? My chest tightened. A large lump formed in my throat as my heart sank. Before I had a chance to break away from the group and go toward the couple, we were whisked into the chapel.

"It's a very serious sin to utter a sound other than a prayer in church. You must stay quiet," someone whispered in my ear as I was beginning to sob. Years later, I did discover that those two people I had seen standing in the corner were indeed my parents. They had come to see how I was adapting, but stayed away from me out of fear it would start another crying spell.

I have no recollection of anything that followed until that evening. I woke up crying in my little bed. The nightlight was shining up on the ceiling. I could see Nicola in his dark blue smock sitting at the foot of my bed.

"Be quiet now. Stop crying. Mom and dad will come tomorrow." He was making this false promise, hoping it would be enough to keep me quiet and help me fall asleep.

My parents didn't come the next day, or any other day for a very long time.

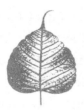

CHAPTER 33

THIS LITTLE GIRL STEALS

The next clear memory I have is of sitting at a long table with at least two pillows under me to gain some height. I still struggled to reach my food. We each wore a white cloth napkin tied around our neck as a bib. The adult in charge of my group sat at the head of the table immediately to my right. She helped me eat when I got teary eyed and tired of feeding myself.

I liked the drinking cups we used. They were made of aluminum so they would not break if dropped. I thought about how nice it would be for my mother to have one. This would make her life so much easier. My little brother could throw it on the floor as many times as he wanted and it would never break, so my mother would not be upset.

I missed my mother so much, I really wanted to make her happy. I did not know how I could possibly take the cup without getting into trouble. One evening at dinner, though, the desire to please my mother became overwhelming. I finished drinking the water from my cup and swiftly put it in my school uniform pocket. It created a bulge, but I was convinced no one could see it. At bedtime, I put the cup in my metal nightstand, thinking how happy I would make my mother when I got to see her again.

I have a clear memory of doing the exact same thing every single day: sitting at a little desk in kindergarten class learning how to count, making shapes with clay, and waiting for the bell to ring for our free play time. Weather permitting, I spent my free playtime running around on the terrace with the other children. I remember the older students fussing over me because I was so little.

Sundays were different. We would get up one half-hour later than during the week, and spend a much longer time in church than usual for the celebration of the Holy Mass. I hated the Holy Mass because it was a reminder that it was visiting day and no one was going to come see me. After Mass came breakfast: a bowl of warm milk with small chunks of bread dunked in it, just like every other day. After breakfast, we would spend most of the day playing games of make-believe, or listening to stories that older blind children read to us from their Braille books.

One rainy Sunday, I remember spending the afternoon in the large dormitory without much to do. I felt particularly sad because I was not going to receive any visitors and they hadn't planned any activities to keep us busy. Children could pretty much do as they pleased as long as they didn't leave the room and didn't talk too loudly. I looked in my metal nightstand to make sure my aluminum cup was still there. Each of us had a metal nightstand next to our bed with a top shelf acting as a seat and the back as a personal towel rack. Between the seat and the top of the metal box was a space for personal decoration. The bottom portion of the stand consisted of a box with a door on the front that could be locked with a padlock if desired.

I was happy to see that the cup was still there. I had nothing else in my nightstand except for my ration of toilet paper. I wondered if the other children had the same things in their nightstands. I decided to crawl under each bed and open the little door to see what was inside. Most of them had toilet paper just like me, but no aluminum cup. When I finished checking the nightstands on my side of the room, I started on the other side.

I was about four or five beds down from the white tent of the group proctor when I discovered a pair of beautiful, soft, fuzzy red boots with rubber soles, lined with sheep's wool. I knew it was sheep's wool because the interior of these boots felt just like the coats of the sheep on the farm. Thinking about sheep made me miss my family even more than usual. I could imagine my little brother being so happy and comfortable wearing those boots. My mother would not have to worry anymore about buying shoes for my brother, and his little feet would always be warm and dry. I had never seen boots like that and I could hardly believe that they existed.

Something came over me. I had to find a way to bring the boots home. For only a split second it felt wrong to take the boots, but immediately I thought to myself that if I took them nobody would ever know that they weren't mine. I took the boots and slid across the space to get to my nightstand as quickly as possible without being seen. I must have looked like a raccoon sliding across the white marble floor with a pair of red boots in my hands.

I stored my treasure in my nightstand, closing the door tightly. Every day I checked to be sure the boots were still there, and touched the fuzzy wool lining that reminded me of home. Having this to look forward to several times a day seemed to make the time away from my family less painful. Now, all that was left to do was wait patiently for my parents to come for me and then everybody would be very happy.

Some days later, the School Director, Miss Antonacci, took an unexpected stroll through the dining room during dinner. Although she lived on the premises, we usually did not see her in the evenings. She was tall, thin, and enviably well-dressed. She wore expensive perfume that wafted ahead of her and lingered as she passed by. Her presence was unmistakable. You could hear her high heels clickity-clacking as she strode across the room. The ambiance in the room changed immediately when she was circulating. A reprimand or a negative comment from the school director was a slap in the face for the staff member in charge and a guaranteed punishment for the student caught in a "sin."

We were required to say, "Good evening, Madame Director," when she approached, but only obliged to stand if asked to do so by a staff member. If Miss Antonacci was escorted by the school principal it was mandatory to stand. As she approached our table, she asked my group custodian, "How are things going with the new little girl?"

The staff member sitting at the head of the table on my right paused for a moment, looked toward her, and replied, "This little girl steals."

Instantly I experienced an ugly new feeling; a big hole opened underneath me and I fell into a dark abyss with nobody to catch me. My magical world full of dreams, fantasy, and naiveté had just been brutally ripped away from me and replaced with shame and humiliation. Until that moment I had no idea that wanting to make my mother's difficult life better could be a mortal sin.

I have no memory of what else was said or how the meal ended, but the bright round tubes of light on the ceiling went dark and nothing anyone did or said could make them bright again. I didn't want to play with the other children anymore. I didn't want to get in line and go to the chapel to recite the evening prayers. I didn't want to climb those wide, cold marble staircases. I didn't want to go through those tall, dark wooden doors that led into the dorm room. I didn't want to count the beds until I reached mine. I didn't want to undress and put on a cold nightgown that didn't smell as if my mother had washed it in fresh water from the stream. I didn't want to say my bedtime prayers. I just wanted my mommy!

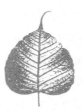

CHAPTER 34

LAST CHRISTMAS ON THE FARM

One day in mid-December, while sitting at my little desk in the kindergarten classroom, I heard what I thought was the sound of bagpipes. Bagpipes were common at religious processions in my community in Basilicata. The teacher suddenly stood and shouted happily, "It's Christmas!" She opened the balcony door and invited us outside, as did all the other classroom teachers on every floor surrounding the interior courtyard. We all listened from our respective balconies to the two bagpipers playing Christmas carols. We clapped and clapped when they finished. My heart leapt with joy because I knew that soon I would be going home.

When the day finally arrived to leave for Christmas vacation, my father came for Nicola and me. We left the school wearing our dress uniforms because we did not own any dress clothes. It was unheard of in those days to go out in public without proper attire. I held my father's right hand and Nicola his left as we walked off the school's premises. We waited across the street to catch the bus that would take us to the train station.

I was so happy to be going home. The raindrops that fell on my face felt like holy water. On the bus, my father told me to hold onto the metal pole for balance and to stay close to him because the bus was very crowded. I did everything he asked me to do because I was so happy.

Getting on the train was very hectic. It was the Christmas rush and many people were traveling with lots of luggage and presents. Even though we didn't have any luggage, my father demanded the right of way because he was traveling with two blind children. Once on the train, we found a compartment where Nicola and I had the window seats. We had fun counting all the things we could see as we sped by: electric poles, trees, houses, tunnels, and the like. I thought how fun it must be to live in a house where you could see the trains going by every day.

The train ride from Naples to Basilicata lasted all day with several changes. When we finally arrived at Castelluccio Inferiore, it was too late to proceed home. We stayed overnight with people my family knew in town.

The next day, as had been scheduled prior to my father's departure, Biagio came to pick us up with the donkey for the last leg of the trip home. Nicola and I were still young enough to ride in the wicker baskets on either side of the donkey, along with other items to counterbalance the weight. We slowly left the modern sounds of the cobblestone streets and moved deeper and deeper into the glorious sounds of the countryside. I filled my lungs with the familiar smells of the vegetation and finally swallowed away the lump that had been lodged in my throat for the past three months. The air, infused with smoke from farmhouses scattered across the hills, enveloped me in a warm blanket of pure joy. The donkey's steady steps kept my basket moving in a gentle rocking motion. Life was sweet again—I was home at last! What a miracle!

When we finally reached the house, the entire family, including Aunt Teodora and her children, were outside waiting in the misty rain. My mother ran toward my basket before the donkey even came to a stop. She hoisted me out and held me tight. She was warm and smelled like love. My father took care of Nicola, and Biagio unsaddled the donkey and took him back to his stall. My mother never put me down until we were inside the house. She had reserved bread-making for the day we arrived so that the house would be extra warm. Hearing the crackling sound of the wood-burning oven, smelling the bread dough rising, and being surrounded by my family was like falling into a well of happiness.

Aunt Teodora held me for a long time. She kissed me over and over. Her face was wet from tears of joy. My sister Maria and my cousins stood around watching bashfully. They didn't know how to approach us now that we had been away at school for so long in a far-away city. We had learned many new things, including how to speak standard Italian. They didn't know whether we would be able to understand them now and could still play with them the way we used to. But as soon as our dress shoes and uniforms came off, the hand-me-downs went back on, and it wasn't long before we picked up our bickering and bouncing around right where we had left off.

On that first day, our mother didn't scold us at all; however, as time went on, she resumed her normal demeanor. One day she threatened to send us back to school early if we didn't stop misbehaving. I didn't take her seriously because I knew very well she would never do that.

I have warm memories of that Christmas. As it turned out, it would be the last one I would spend on the farm. Every night after dinner, we all gathered around the fire to keep warm until bedtime. Some evenings my parents would make popcorn in a pan over the fire. Some nights, we would savor my mother's delicious *chiulini*, a ravioli-shaped pastry filled with chestnut puree and cocoa.

Whenever we sat in a semicircle around the fire, my youngest blind sibling, two-year-old Pietro, liked to make his rounds from one end of the semicircle to the other, identifying each person by touching their knees. Sometimes we would switch places to play tricks on him and he would get a big kick out of identifying the person correctly.

One such evening, as we were playing this game, Biagio mistakenly stretched his legs at the wrong moment, causing little Pietro to trip and fall into the fire. He was pulled out almost instantly as he fell in, but the damage was done. The sense of guilt saddled Biagio's soul and lives with him to this day. The burn scars still mark Pietro's bottom. Growing up, I remember my mother referring to this incident as one of the many reasons she pushed so hard to leave the farm.

The best part of the Christmas holiday was the celebration of Epiphany on January 6th. That was when the old, ragged lady came down the chimney during the night to leave candy or coal in the children's stockings, depending on their behavior during the past year. Although

I always looked forward to Epiphany, this time things were different. A sick feeling settled in my stomach as the day grew near. Sadly I knew that the blissful time I was having at home was coming to an end. Immediately after the celebration of my favorite holiday, I would have to say goodbye to my family again and return to school.

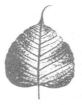

CHAPTER 35

UNCLE FEDELE LEAVES FOR AMERICA

Unlike my first journey to the school, I knew now what was waiting for me. I spent every minute agonizing—anticipating the painful separation from my parents that I would soon have to face. "You're a big girl now," my parents would say. "You shouldn't cry anymore." As if it were that easy.

The journey was memorable for another reason. It coincided with my Uncle Fedele's departure for America. He was one of my mother's youngest brothers and had been born in New York. The four of us, my parents, Nicola and I, were part of the entourage of relatives escorting him to the port of Naples where he would board a ship that would take him across the Atlantic.

Our trip was long and tiresome, and we used a variety of vehicles to reach Naples. One thing I'll never forget was my first ride in an automobile. It was stuffed with as many people as it could possibly hold. I remember being squeezed in the backseat on my father's knees. There was barely enough room to breathe, but it was exciting to be inside a small box that moved so fast. Outside it was dark and rainy, and I knew that if I had been riding a donkey, I would be soaking wet.

We must have spent the first night with a family in Naples. The next morning after I was dressed and ready to go, I remember looking around the room. A large balcony brought in lots of light. A glass door led into another room exactly like ours. It also had a big balcony with lots of light.

When I approached the glass door, a little girl from the other room approached it as well, facing me. She was exactly my height, so I wanted to meet her and play with her. At one point my mother walked over to me, and a woman in the other room approached the little girl at the same time. When my mother walked away from me and the other little girl's mother backed away from her, I decided to open the door. When I looked around the door there was no little girl. I quickly closed the door and again the little girl was facing me from the other side. I opened the door again but there was no little girl. I was so confused. Finally my mother stopped laughing, "That's you in the glass door. It's called a mirror, Carmelina." My mother's explanation didn't solve the mystery for me. I continued opening and closing that door trying to find that little girl.

That afternoon at the port we joined a crowd of many families saying goodbye to loved ones who were departing. The mood was somber. I could hear some people crying. Moment by moment, the time for the ship to sail neared. In the mid-1950s, the prospect of reuniting with emigrating family members was remote. This profound sadness was compounded by the recent tragedy of the *Andrea Doria*, a vessel full of Italian immigrants heading to New York that had sunk off the coast of Massachusetts. Uncle Fedele had been scheduled to travel on the *Andrea Doria*, but his departure date was changed at the last minute for some reason. We all felt blessed by a miracle but apprehensive nonetheless.

I stood next to my mother and held her hand while we all waited for the dreadful moment. She repeatedly wished my uncle a safe trip and sent her love and good wishes to all the relatives in New York. "If God is willing, maybe one day we will see each other again." Then she broke down in tears and so did everyone else.

The passengers stood with their families until the very last possible second before boarding. When the final call came a flurry of embraces and tears erupted. Once they were on board there was a long wait, long enough for everyone to regain composure. When the crowd spotted the passengers emerging on deck they exploded in cheers, and family members on both the shore and the ship frantically waved handkerchiefs. When my mother heard the first blast of the ship's horn announcing its imminent departure, she put a handkerchief in my right hand and lifted me onto my father's shoulders. "You are wearing a red dress. Maybe Uncle Fedele will be able to spot you among the crowd," she said as she wiped away her tears. I waved that handkerchief for what seemed to be forever.

The ship slowly and gently moved away from the dock. The crowd remained immobile and silent for some moments as though hypnotized until the vessel finally disappeared from sight.

In his first letter to my mother, Uncle Fedele wrote, "I felt luckier than the other passengers on deck waving our last goodbyes to the families on shore, because I knew exactly where to throw my kisses. I could see Carmelina towering above the crowd in her pretty red dress, waving the handkerchief. I felt proud in so many ways but I really sobbed when she became a small red dot that blended into the beautiful coast of Naples. I wished it did not have to be this way."

Later that day, Nicola and I arrived at the residential School for the Blind. I have no clear recollection of the trip. It must have been late in the evening and I must have been sleeping. I do remember being carried upstairs fireman-style by a staff member already in her nightgown. Everything was dark and quiet. I wasn't wearing shoes. I felt tricked and abandoned by my parents. The lump in my throat was back and I just couldn't swallow it away. I started crying and screaming for my mother. The staff member told me to stop crying, "You are a big girl now and big girls don't cry. Everyone else is sleeping quietly. Now you do the same." She dropped me into a cold bed, pulled the covers over me, and walked away.

CHAPTER 36

A LESSON IN FORGIVENESS

S ome of the children came back from the holidays with new toys. A boy sitting close to me in the kindergarten classroom had received a beautiful harmonica for Christmas. I was extremely envious. I had a plastic watch. It didn't do anything but sit on my wrist and be plasticky. With the harmonica, on the other hand, you could make beautiful sounds. When I saw the other children's toys, I didn't like my watch at all anymore. It was unfair. I asked the boy with the harmonica if he wanted to exchange toys for one day. Much to my surprise, he accepted right away.

The harmonica was smooth and heavy and I felt important holding it in my hand. I couldn't believe how lucky some children were to receive such beautiful gifts. I couldn't wait for class to be over so I could play it, and I played it as often as I could throughout the day. It didn't seem real to me to hold such an expensive toy.

The next morning, I got ready as quickly as possible so that I could play it some more before I had to give it up. I went out onto the balcony and while I was playing, the beautiful harmonica slipped out of my hands and fell into the construction site two stories below.

My heart sank. *What am I going to do now? What will I tell the boy?* He was going to be angry and hate me. Everybody was going to be angry and hate me. I was going to receive a serious punishment. The teacher was going to write to my parents and ask them to reimburse the cost of the harmonica. My parents were going to be sad because they didn't have the money. And I was going to be sad for the rest of my life, and it was entirely my fault! I wished I had fallen into the construction site along with the harmonica. At least I wouldn't have to face the little boy and make him sad. I prayed to God to make the harmonica appear in my pocket, but God seemed not to hear me.

The dreadful moment to go into my kindergarten class and face the inevitable came in a flash. I didn't want to face little Tomassino, but he approached my desk in a hurry, holding my plastic watch in his right hand. "Here's your watch, Carmelina, can I have my harmonica back?" I sat paralyzed in my chair at his words. I prayed and implored God to make Tomassino want to keep my plastic watch. I didn't want to tell him the truth. And then I cried, but to no avail. He asked for his harmonica again.

The teacher intervened. "What is the matter, Carmelina?" The time had come and I had to confess the whole story. Tomassino was sad to hear the fate of his harmonica, but I cried even harder when I heard him say, "It's OK. I forgive you." I didn't know whether he did that because he was just a nice boy or as a result of all the intensive religious teachings we received. Whatever it was, it certainly saved my skin and taught me an important lesson: it is possible to forgive and be forgiven for a mistake that might seem to be unforgivable.

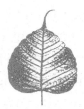

CHAPTER 37

MAKING ESPRESSO IN KINDERGARTEN

The school routine was so similar from day to day that only very happy or sad times stayed in my memory. We got into the same boring uniform each morning, repeated the same prayers, ate the same miserly breakfast, spent all morning sitting at a desk, always afraid of doing or saying the wrong thing and getting punished for it. Never anything fun to look forward to. It felt like an endless boring existence with no relief in sight.

When it rained, I felt extra sad in fear that the rain would wash away the family house on the farm with my family in it, and I would be left alone and sad for the rest of my life. I felt like I was in a prison for children, but what kind of crime had I committed? Was being born blind a crime?

Sundays were exceptionally painful as we spent hour after hour waiting for the phone to ring. That's how children were summoned to the visiting room when their family members arrived. For some of us, the phone never rang. Occasionally some generous parents would bring an extra box of cookies for their child to share with his or her friends. That was always a bright moment, but bittersweet because I always wished that those cookies had come from my parents.

One day the predictable routine changed. The kindergarten teacher brought an electric hot plate and a stovetop espresso coffeepot to class.

"Today, we're going to learn to make coffee," she said. "In modern life now, we don't need to be in a kitchen anymore to make coffee." She showed us all the pieces of the coffeepot and demonstrated how to fill up the bottom with water, the middle basket with coffee, and to screw the top on tightly so that when the water started boiling, the steam would move up through the coffee grounds and shoot into the upper part as coffee. She showed us how to plug in the hot plate and put the pot on it.

"You must always put the coffee pot in the center of the burner. As the hot plate warms up, you can feel the heat evenly distributed around the coffeepot as it gets hotter and hotter. Make sure that you listen for the gurgling sound that tells you when the coffee is almost ready," she said. "As soon as the sound stops, you have to remove the coffee pot from the burner otherwise you can burn the coffee."

She poured the coffee into a paper cup and went around the room so that we could each have a sniff or a small taste. When she got to me, the coffee smelled so good I was disappointed that I could only have a little sniff. I wished I were the teacher so I could drink a whole cup.

Her idea of show-and-tell was brilliant for a teacher of visually impaired children, but it almost turned into a fire disaster. She set the hot plate on top of a small desk and it became completely scorched. She made sure we all got to feel the burned little table so that we would remember the important lesson as we got older: to be very careful with heat when cooking, while not implying it would be unsafe for blind people to learn to cook.

I don't know how dedicated a teacher she really was, or how important it was for five and six-year-olds to watch an adult make coffee, but for me this lesson was such a fun experience that I put the little burner and the little coffeepot in my imaginary dream house for when I would be a grown up, along with all the fancy toys I had seen certain rich kids play with. I would also have a typewriter, a telephone, and, of course, my little car without a roof, and loads and loads of chocolate everywhere. I had lots of fun in my dream house. I escaped into it every waking moment when I was not required to pay attention to something else.

CHAPTER 38

CALLED TO THE DIRECTOR'S OFFICE

Ninety-one days waited before we could go home again for our Easter break. We all counted the days. Sometimes when I tried to imagine how long it would take for ninety-one days to go by, I felt sick to my stomach. I wished I could have a nice toy to play with so that I would feel better.

Slowly and painfully, the ninety-one days ticked by and we began planning the celebrations for Fat Tuesday or Mardi Gras. A welcome break in an otherwise gloomy existence, we talked about Mardi Gras for days before it was actually upon us. Mardi Gras preceded Ash Wednesday, the first day of Lent, which lasted forty days until Easter Sunday.

On the day of Mardi Gras, we had only two hours of class, very informal, and we spent the rest of the day playing or finding ways to disguise ourselves. I was the youngest child in the school so the older girls had lots of fun deciding how to dress me up as a princess. They had no material to work with, so they took a bedspread, wrapped it around me, and made various knots so that it would look like a long dress. They made a tiara with a piece of Braille paper that they cut, folded, and stapled together.

"How pretty you look!" said our staff member as she came out of her tent. "How ingenious it was to come up with such a costume just by tying knots and using safety pins!" I felt ecstatic that she and the older girls were fussing over me so much.

As soon as the lunch bell rang, we all hurried to get to our spot in line. The no-talking rule was not enforced on this day. The joyful mood throughout the school was overwhelming. A real feast waited for us in the dining room. First course: baked lasagna, followed by sausages and an assortment of pickled vegetables. Then seasonal fruits, followed by a *sanguinaccio*, the traditional Mardi Gras dessert that used to be made with pig's blood, plus chocolate, candied fruit, sugar, and spices, but was now made without the pig's blood. A drop of wine and a drop of coffee sealed the meal.

We spent the afternoon playing games, singing, and trying to guess the identities of older students who had ingeniously created masks with Braille paper and were wearing costumes they had fashioned from bedding and odd bits of clothing.

The normal routine resumed at 7:30 p.m. with the mandatory half-hour evening prayer in the chapel, followed by dinner and then bed. This was the time of day most difficult for me when I would start thinking about my family. The next day would be Ash Wednesday which meant that in fewer than 40 days I would be going home.

Spring slowly arrived. As the temperature grew warmer, we began shedding layers of underclothing: first the wool dress that we wore just underneath our blue-and-white smock uniform, and then the thermal sweater, leaving just a slip and underwear under the smock. Feeling lighter was a pleasant sensation.

Easter was almost upon us and I was happy. One day our group leader escorted me into Miss Antonacci's office. A student was taken to the director's office for only two reasons: either something really bad had happened, or something really good was about to happen. In my case, something really bad was about to happen.

"Carmelina, we received a letter from your parents. Unfortunately, they will not be able to come for you this Easter. You and Nicola will be spending the holiday here along with a few other children who cannot go home either." She explained that the vacation was just too short and expensive for my family to make the trip twice in less than a week.

I thought I had already experienced the feeling of the floor disappearing from under my feet, but it felt even worse this time. I hated being sad, I hated to be away from my family, I hated everything!

I just wanted to go home and be with my family like everybody else. I wanted to be happy but I just couldn't.

On the Tuesday before Easter, one by one almost all of the children were picked up by their parents and left the school. Although I knew I was not going anywhere, I still hoped that a mistake had been made and that somehow my parents would come for me and for my brother. I must have spent the rest of the week in some kind of a trance in order to get through such a lonely time, because I have no recollection of anything that happened during those few days.

As soon as school was back in session we calculated that there would be fewer than sixty days before we would go home for the long summer vacation of four months. From that moment on, every time I felt sad I quickly thought of the four months I would soon be spending with my family and that made me feel better. During recreation time to make the days feel like they were going by faster, we often talked about all of the fun things we were going to do with our families during the summer.

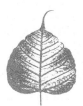

CHAPTER 39

AN OUTBREAK OF MEASLES

Toward the middle of May, a measles epidemic broke out. It seemed as if every day several children were whisked away to the infirmary where they were quarantined until the ambulance came to transport them to the hospital. Whenever we had a chance to talk among ourselves, we became defiant.

"Oh no," one of my friends would say, "I am not going to the hospital! If I come down with the measles, when they put me in the ambulance, I'll break the window and just jump out."

"Me too," I would reply.

"I'll run away from the infirmary in the middle of the night," someone else would add. All of us seemed to have a clear plan as to what we would do if we came down with the disease. Within a few days a staff member approached me, took a quick look at my face, and immediately escorted me to the infirmary. Within a few hours, I was in an ambulance on my way to the hospital. Once in the ambulance, I thought about the plans we had all made about breaking the window and jumping out, but the best I could do was to touch the window with my index finger.

At the hospital my bed was placed in a hallway surrounded by doors; this would be my room for the next month, the duration of my stay. A nurse handed me a cable with a button on the end that I could push if I needed anything and then walked away. I could hear faint voices from the other side of the wall, followed by an occasional thump. From the adjacent rooms, I could hear noises, but couldn't decipher any specifics. After some time, I pushed the button because I needed to use the bathroom. I pushed and pushed but nobody came, and finally my bladder gave out and I wet the bed. I lay there crying in my wet bed for hours. When a nurse finally came, she hoisted me out of bed and replaced the sheets with a plastic liner.

Before they served dinner, somebody from the adjacent room opened the door.

"Is someone there?" she shouted. I recognized her voice. She was from my school.

"Carmelina," I replied, with a little delight in my voice.

"Oh, Carmelina, you just came in today, right? There are some other girls from the school here," she said, "and there are also some boys who are all together in one big room on the other side of the wall. They'll be serving dinner soon. The food is pretty disgusting, but at least here nobody forces you to eat it." I was relieved to hear that.

Within a few days, we all became well enough to be allowed out of bed. There wasn't much supervision so we could move about freely in the immediate surroundings. It felt strange to go from such a strict and authoritarian environment to having practically no rules at all. We became friends with some other patients in the adjacent rooms. They were older people convalescing from various diseases, and they were shocked to see so many young, blind kids alone in the hospital. They occasionally gave us some guidance and reassurances to help us tolerate being there all by ourselves.

One day we girls ventured out to visit the boys' room. Their door was open and we heard lots of chaos going on. It was a large room with about seven or eight beds. The boy occupying the bed on the opposite side of the wall from my bed would kick his legs up in the air. On the way down, he would hit his heels against the wall. That explained the thumping noise I kept hearing over and over when I was in bed. When I finally heard his voice above all of the chaos, I recognized him; it was my brother Nicola! Suddenly I didn't feel quite so lonely and abandoned anymore.

Nicola was eight years old, sharing the room with other blind boys from the school; some were his age and some younger. He and his roommates acted as though they were in control of the situation. They always knew what day it was and how many days we had been in the hospital. They also predicted how many more days we would be there.

The boys' room quickly became the entertainment room for the whole section of the floor. The boys would split themselves into two teams, one called the right side (of the room), and the other the left side. Each person would take a turn as the goalkeeper for his team. Each team tried to score a goal by hitting the opposite wall with a pillow while the goalkeeper tried to catch the pillow before it hit the wall. With most of these blind players having extra sharp hearing it was nearly impossible for anyone to get away with cheating.

The boys bounced around the room as though the beds were trampolines. This game would go on for hours and was fun to watch. The hospital staff members were amazed at how the blind kids could jump around the room as they did without missing a step. I enjoyed watching too, but what I really wanted was to play with them.

On the girls' side, we couldn't do anything like that. For one thing, we didn't have the same setup or the space that they had. But more to the point, girls were just not supposed to roughhouse like that. Even with lack of supervision, we still observed some of the strict rules instilled in us at the School for the Blind, including this one: beyond kindergarten, girls and boys don't mix.

At meal times, the older children would immediately announce what was on the tray. We all got excited or disgusted over the same foods. We got disgusted over soup with cheese that would stick to your spoon; we got excited when it was just a glass of milk with Melba toast and orange marmalade. In the mid-1950s, many people in Southern Italy were very poor. Eating bread with jam in the morning or any other time of the day was very uncommon because sugar was so expensive; therefore, we considered orange marmalade a real treat.

On Sundays, some of the older patients would take us to Mass, which was held in a large open space in the hospital. I never looked forward to Mass because I had to remain still and quiet for a long time, and that made me feel sad and lonely. One day after Mass, they took us onto a terrace where we could see people sitting on balconies across the courtyard on the floors above. An older gentleman at one point said to me, "Can you see people sitting over there on that balcony?"

"Yes, a little bit."

"That is the isolation unit for people who have typhoid."

I had heard that typhoid was a deadly disease! Did that mean the people that I was looking at were going to die? I quickly looked away and tried to stop thinking about it. Death scared me.

Occasionally one of the students from our group got to leave the hospital and go back to school. The hospital staff never gave us any information as to why that particular student was leaving and not others, so we just waited and waited, continued playing games, and continued guessing as to when we would leave.

One day I wandered into a nearby empty room. I noticed that there was a balcony. I looked outside. I could see the landing, but not a railing. I finally decided to venture out there. I got on my hands and knees to make sure that I inched my way to the edge slowly, just in case there was no railing. When I got to the edge, I raised my right hand upward and touched a railing! The reason I could not see it was because the metal rods were very thin and did not provide enough contrast with the walls of the building on the other side. It felt good to be on the balcony. It was quiet. The air was fresh. There was no one around to bark orders at me. I was happy. I sat on the cool floor and began to think about my family. The farm. The animals.

CHAPTER 40

BRIEF CONVERSATION WITH MAJOR CONSEQUENCES

One day, the announcement finally came that we were all going home. It didn't really mean we were going home-home, just that we were leaving the hospital to return to the residential School for the Blind.

We didn't get a chance to ride in motor vehicles very often, so the trip back in the van was a treat. School was already out for the year and the staff had waited to bring us back to avoid contaminating the other children. We were relieved to finally be out of the hospital and soon to be reunited with our families. Our parents had been notified by telegram when to pick us up.

One afternoon while playing outside, I could feel my parents' presence. Within minutes I heard their voices several yards away. I wanted to run up to them but I had to respect protocol. They were expected to greet Miss Antonacci the school director, and other staff members before they could come to me. During that brief conversation, the director said something to my mother that wounded her for the rest of her life. Referring to the Easter holiday, she said, "It must have taken a lot of courage to spend the holidays without your children."

I don't know whether the remark was genuine or whether it was meant to be mean-spirited, but my mother took great offense and was never able to come to terms with it. During the train ride back home, my mother told my father, "I don't care what we have to do—lie, cheat, or steal—within the next year we are moving to Naples to be near the school. I'm never going to live away from my children again."

CHAPTER 41

LAST SUMMER ON THE FARM

In spite of all of the hard work in the summer to deal with all the harvests, my mother ordered my father to go to Naples on several occasions until he came home with a plan: a house for us to live in and prospects for a job. I noticed that things were hustling and bustling more than usual in our small farmhouse. Preparations for leaving the farm were mixed in with the usual dawn to dusk hard work.

One day, a tailor came to the house with fabric samples. He measured my father for a suit. On another occasion, someone came to collect wool from the sheep in order to make mattresses and quilts for the city life that we were about to begin. My parents started selling all of the livestock so that they could have money to buy furniture and other necessities for the rented apartment in Naples. The long-term plan was to rent our farm to Aunt Teodora and her family.

I spent most of the time at my mother's side helping her with her chores. She promised to give me a ten *lira* coin at the end of the summer if I behaved and helped her as much as I could. I had never owned money before, so I was very excited. I wanted to please my mother so I followed her orders. At the end of the summer I got my coin, which was enough to buy two pieces of hard candy.

One afternoon, before my father was due to leave on one of his numerous trips to Naples, I heard them talking in the kitchen about the move. I was sitting on the doorstep enjoying my favorite snack, a slice of homemade bread and some sheep's milk cheese. My mother sounded somewhat distraught and impatient with my father for not finding a job prospect.

"What do you expect me to do?" asked my father. "I can't invent a job. I'm a farmer. I'm not qualified to do anything in the city."

My father was not as eager to move to Naples as my mother. He always tried to come up with a good reason to delay the process and this infuriated her.

"Maybe the kids have a little more vision than we think" my father said. "As they get a little older they probably won't mind being away from us, and when they come home during the summer, I'm sure they will have fun doing chores around the farm."

"We've discussed this already and it's not going to work," said my mother.

"Remember last night, when Carmelina was pointing at the moon? That to me means that she can see quite a bit."

At the sound of that, my mother lost all patience and unleashed the accusations that she had avoided expressing for many years. "You just can't help but be your usual stupid, stubborn self, can you?" she shouted with an angry, teary voice, "If you didn't want to have blind children, you should have been more cautious in bed instead of acting like a dog in heat. How much vision do you think it takes for someone to locate a big bright dot in the middle of a black sky? She can see the moon, but she'll never be able to see the stars," she sobbed, burying her face in a tea towel.

My father stormed out of the house, nearly tripping over me on the doorstep. It was the first time I had witnessed an argument of this caliber between my parents. I was petrified. I thought my mother was going to cry so hard that she would die and my father would never come back home. I felt helpless, guilty, sad, and afraid. I began to cry.

CHAPTER 42

LEARNING TO READ AND WRITE

The end of the summer meant going back to school for Nicola and me. This time we were a little less heartsick than the previous year because our mother had promised us that by Christmas the family would be living in the same city as us. I looked forward to sharing that wonderful news with my friends at school.

Monday through Saturday the school day started at 8:30 a.m. for academic classes. One o'clock was lunch; 1:30 p.m. to 2:30 p.m. free time; 2:30 p.m. to 3:30 p.m. knitting; 3:30 p.m. to 4:30 p.m. music; 4:30 p.m. to 5:00 p.m. free time; 5:00 p.m. to 7:30 p.m. homework; 7:30 p.m. to 8:00 p.m. chapel; 8:00 p.m. dinner; 9:30 p.m. lights out.

On Sundays, instead of rising at 6:30 a.m., we were allowed to sleep until 7:00 a.m. Mass was at 8:00 a.m., followed by breakfast and free time until 10:00 a.m.; 10:00 a.m. to 12:00 p.m. was homework, followed by lunch at 1:00 p.m. We spent the rest of the afternoon being bored, or for the lucky ones, visits with family from home. The routine never changed. There never seemed to be a good day for me at this school and Sundays were particularly bad. But I comforted myself by thinking about how soon my whole family would be moving to Naples, and then I too would have visitors every Sunday.

In first grade, crying and being sad was no longer an option. "You're a big girl now. You don't have time to cry anymore. This is where learning becomes serious," they told me. And so it did. First grade seemed so much harder than kindergarten. No more sculpting with clay, playing with building blocks, or counting colorful balls. Now we had to remain longer in our seats and learn all kinds of important things, including all the tools that blind students used at that time in Italy.

The first grade teacher gave us a general overview of all the things we would be learning in the next five years. She first let us explore two large raised relief maps hanging on the wall. The first one was the Italian peninsula in the shape of a boot. It was so tall that I could hardly reach the top. The map was exceptionally well detailed. It included indentations for every gulf, a raised line for every river, and a small or large dot for every city, depending on its size. Every mountain range and lake was detailed with extreme accuracy and scaled to size. The second map represented the entire continent of Europe.

In the corner, all by itself, stood a very large raised relief globe of the world. The teacher gave it a spin and said, "By the end of fifth grade you will know the name of every country, every big city, every mountain range, every important river, every ocean, and every important lake in the entire world." I felt scared. *Will I be able to learn all of these things? I will have to do a lot of work and all of it by myself, without my parents. I wish I were the teacher. She already knows everything.*

After our tour of the classroom, we returned to our seats to become familiar with all the writing tools that blind people in Italy used in the 1950s. She gave us each a Braille slate and a stylus. I liked having my own Braille slate. It wasn't exactly a fun toy, but it made me feel important and a little bit like a grown-up.

The slate was a 9 by 11-inch aluminum plate etched with horizontal grooves. It had a half-inch wide open frame attached by hinges at the top. I would open the frame and insert a piece of stiff paper. Once I closed the frame, pins on the sides of the aluminum plate would hold the sheet of paper in place. The frame had holes on either side, evenly spaced from top to bottom, representing the number of lines that could fit on the page. A separate horizontal guide with pegs on either end would rest securely in the holes representing the lines. I could move the guide all the way down the page as I wrote.

The guide had two horizontal lines of cells, each cell having spaces for six dots: dots 1, 2, and 3 vertically on the right and 4, 5, and 6 vertically on the left. In each cell I could compose a Braille letter which was a variable combination of the six dots.

I would create these letters with a special stylus that I would hold firmly by curling my index finger around the top and stabilizing the stylus with my thumb and the first knuckle of my middle finger. Then, I would apply pressure on any of the six positions within the cell, pushing the paper into the horizontal grooves in the aluminum plate and creating an embossed letter. For example, the letter "a" is one dot in the upper right corner of the cell. The letter "b" is a dot in the top right corner plus a dot in the middle right. The letter "c" is a dot in the top right corner, and a dot in the top left corner. The letter "d" is top right, top left, and middle left.

I had to compose the Braille words from right to left so that when I was finished writing, I could open the frame, flip the page and read the embossed words with my fingers, from left to right. By removing the guide from the frame, I suddenly had a 9 by 11-inch surface to make embossed drawings.

"You will learn to draw subjects using templates that you hold firmly on the page, using your stylus to emboss dots all around the perimeter of the template," the teacher said. "When you are finished, you flip the page and compare the template to your Braille drawing to see how accurately you did it."

She explained that over the years we would learn to draw an object on the Ballu slate without the template for reference. She'd tell us, "This is a skill that you must master in order to pass the state-issued fifth grade exam. For the exam you will have to draw an object perfectly enough so that anyone who sees it or feels it can successfully identify it. And you will have to draw it without a template."

She gave us each a template to identify before we started embossing. Some were holding a butterfly, some a vase with flowers. I was holding a dog. When it was my turn to identify my template, I was already crying.

"Why are you crying, Carmelina?" the teacher asked me. I couldn't tell her why I was crying. The template reminded me of our dog on the farm with my family, and I wanted to be there too. She felt my forehead, wondering if I had a fever.

"Would you like to go to the infirmary? Do you feel sick?" I couldn't answer her. "If you are not going to answer me, then you have to stop crying."

I took my handkerchief out of my left pocket, wiped away my tears and blew my nose. I started pushing dots around the perimeter of a little dog with its tail sticking up.

"Once you are in third grade you will have to learn to use the Ballu and Regolo slates. With the Ballu slate your drawings can be much more refined, and with the Regolo slate you will be able to print letters just like a sighted person," our teacher said. "Although you won't use these slates until you are in third grade, I still would like you to be familiar with them."

Drawing and hand-lettering were skills required on state exams for both sighted and blind students. Therefore, drawing and hand-lettering would be mandatory parts of our curriculum throughout grade school. To develop this skill we would use the Ballu slate. It was larger in size, and we would use a much sharper stylus with it because the grooves were much closer together.

With this slate we could generate tactile print letters also by writing from right to left. The guide for the Ballu slate had three rows of cells. The middle row was used to emboss the lower case letters, such as "a" or "c." The cells above and below were used to create extensions above or below the middle. For example, the extension below for the lower case "g" or the extension above for the upper case "L." Once you flipped the page, the embossed letters could be read from left to right by either a blind or sighted person.

The Ballu slate was also crucial for drawing. Using a stylus in freehand mode we could create tactile diagrams. Because the grooves or etchings in the Ballu plate were finer and closer together than those in the regular Braille slate, we could create fine lines that felt like embroidery. We would start by using templates similar to cookie cutters. But by the end of fifth grade, when we were subjected to a state exam, we would be required to produce a fairly elaborate drawing without a template.

The final tool we had to master was the Regolo slate. The aluminum plate of this slate was totally smooth with no grooves or etching, but it allowed us to print with a pencil or ball-point pen just like sighted people; from left to right, without embossing. We would draw each letter within the rectangular cell that moved along as each letter was written. It was also a much faster writing method than the Ballu slate.

With a Regolo slate you inserted the paper in the same manner used for the other two slates. It had a line guide with one cell and two pull-levers that you could manipulate when you needed room for extended letters, such as the lower case "p," or any capital letter. After each letter, you would move the mechanism one click over and write the next letter. At the end of each line, you simply pushed the mechanism all the way to the left and moved the guide down the page, one line at a time. Unlike the Ballu and Braille slates, this form of writing left no tactile traces for a blind reader. However, it was perfect for writing to sighted people. This was the only skill we learned with a sighted assistant in the classroom.

When it came to learning math, we used small metal pegs, each with a tactile Roman number or arithmetic symbol embossed on the top. The pegs were stored in a rectangular wooden box with three rows of compartments. Each smaller compartment contained several pegs of the same number. For example, the first smaller box held ten pegs with the number "1" embossed on them. The lid of the box contained a metal grid with holes into which the pegs fit. We could assemble a math problem by placing the number pegs as well as the math operators in the correct sequence and then proceed to solve the equation, posting the answer in the grid, one line below. Visually, this looked exactly the same as a math problem on paper for sighted students.

Our teachers believed it was imperative that blind students learn to conceptualize the visual world, that is, to know how things looked and felt. They wanted us to grow up with a rich and descriptive vocabulary that would serve us well in the sighted world.

"The playing field is not level," they would constantly tell us.

"You always have to keep several steps ahead of everybody else if you want to be an active participant in society."

This line of thinking was convincing to us because all of our classroom teachers were blind themselves. They had first-hand experience.

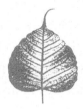

CHAPTER 43

SUNDAY VISITS, CHRISTMAS IN NAPLES, FIRST COMMUNION, PIANO LESSONS

Poverty was still running rampant in Southern Italy in the mid-1950s and for most households a telephone line was financially out of reach. As a result we had no direct contact with our parents unless they came to visit us at the school. I knew my family was supposed to move to Naples, but I had no way of knowing when that would happen. Nevertheless, every Sunday I was on pins and needles hoping this would be the day I would finally get called to the visiting room.

One gloomy Sunday afternoon, while playing silly games and being bored, the call for me finally came. The staff member who answered the only extension on the floor called out, "Cantisani, you have visitors!" My heart leaped. I hoped this meant my parents had moved to Naples and this would be the first Sunday of many more to come when I would have visitors like most of the other children.

I felt wobbly when I got out of my desk chair. I walked down the stairs floating on a cloud. I could hear voices coming from the visiting room and I could smell the outside world. As I entered, a woman from the right corner of the room started walking toward me. She wore a raincoat that made a swishy noise and her shoes made a clickety-clack sound on the marble floor with each step. She called out my name. It was my mother! She kissed me on both cheeks. My father kissed me as well. His face was smooth but his mustache poked me a little on my cheek.

Nicola was sitting with my parents when I arrived. I was jealous that he had already spent more time with them than I had.

"We live here now. We kept our promise. Are you happy?" my father asked.

That was music to my ears and comforting to my heart and soul. I had been waiting so long for this day. I was so overwhelmed with emotions that I became shy and couldn't speak.

"We'll be coming to visit you every Sunday from now on," said my mother as I sat down next to her.

Everything we did or said with our parents was on full display in the visiting room. A staff member sat at a desk kitty-corner from where my family and I were sitting. That made me uncomfortable and I wondered why we needed to be so closely scrutinized in this setting.

Our visitors had no privacy. In fact, based on the noises I could hear coming from each family group, I could tell what kind of treats they were unwrapping. The more expensive treats such as cookies, chocolates, and candies always made more enticing noises while they were unwrapped. Families of modest means like mine brought seasonal fruit wrapped in newspaper. At the time, a box of cookies cost more than a loaf of bread. With three blind kids there was no way my family could afford to bring such treats. I wished I could prevent my parents from feeling bad about that. All that mattered to me was being with my family at last.

My mother smelled different now. Her hair was short and permed. Her hands no longer carried the aroma of homemade bread and fresh vegetables. She tried to carry herself with the sophistication of a city person now that she was living in Naples, but I could feel her insecurity. She looked around every time she moved or talked hoping for acceptance, but fearing disapproving glances from the staff and the other parents. City-dwellers were very judgmental of country folk and considered them to be peasants.

Without her support system from the farm community she was really at a loss. She spoke softly to hide the fact that she didn't speak standard Italian very well. I wished I could make things better for her. Nevertheless, I was euphoric that my family was now close and I could look forward to a happier future. Perhaps there would be a happier future for my mother, too, because every Sunday she would see other parents with blind children and realize she was not alone.

"Next Sunday we will be here again," my father said proudly.

"And when you come home for Christmas it will only take two bus rides, and in a little over an hour you'll be home!" added my mother.

My heart swelled with joy. I couldn't wait to see our new house so close to the school. Knowing that from now on I would only need to wait six days between visits, made everything more tolerable. I just couldn't wait until Christmas!

With lots of hope, many prayers, and an enormous amount of patience, we made it to Christmas. My father picked up Nicola and me toward the end of departure day. After two bus rides we walked the half mile or so from the bus stop to our new house. Along the way we passed crowds of people and I heard street vendors shouting out what they were selling. This was new and exciting for us. The cobblestone paved streets were narrow and I could smell different aromas emanating from each doorway. I kept thinking about what our new apartment was going to be like.

"People are noticing how smart you look in your dress uniforms," my father said to Nicola and me. I walked a little taller after he said that.

It was already dark when we reached our building. It was built monastery style, like most of the buildings in the neighborhood. We entered the courtyard through an archway. Except for the two-story building opposite the archway, every other structure was at ground level. The courtyard was muddy and I was afraid I would ruin my dress shoes. We walked up an outdoor staircase of eight steps to a landing, then left, and up nineteen more. On the second landing, we turned left and walked down a long covered walkway with a railing on the left. We passed two entrances leading to rooms the landlord used in addition to the entire bottom floor. At the very end of the long walkway was a small enclosed porch with a door on the right that opened into our kitchen.

When we entered our apartment, my mother, Maria, Biagio, and my youngest brother Pietro, were all waiting for us with open arms. The house smelled really, really good. My mother had made a meat sauce with bones she had purchased from the local butcher. We now had a three-burner stove with a propane tank. I was happy that my mother no longer had to work so hard at getting the wood fire going in order to cook anything. We were living in the city now, and life was much easier than on the farm.

"Cooking with propane is certainly convenient, but it's very expensive, and we have to make sure we don't run out of propane when the stores are closed," said my mother. "For now, we don't have an oven so we'll have to get through Christmas without our favorite treats and of course, no more homemade bread."

After dinner my mother showed us around the apartment. We had new furniture, nothing rustic like on the farm. Everything was smooth and light. The kitchen was a large room that had been separated by a partition. On the dining area side, there was a twin bed where my oldest brother Biagio slept, in addition to the table. In the bedroom, I would be sharing a twin bed with my sister, and Nicola would sleep across the bottom half of the big bed where my parents and Pietro slept.

The last thing our mother showed us was our very first Christmas tree ever. She had decorated it with colorful balls, gold and silver streamers, lights, and a thin veil of snow that draped over the branches.

"You have to feel it very, very gently," my mother would say. "Otherwise you will poke holes in the veil of snow and it won't look pretty anymore."

She allowed us to gently touch one ornament and said, "There are many more like this away from the edge and they are all made of chocolate. If you behave you will be able to eat them on Epiphany Day."

Suddenly, she plugged the tree into the wall and we could see the blazing lights. My siblings and I marveled at the tree. It was great living in the city and having all these wonderful things.

"We can't leave it plugged in for too long, because electricity is very expensive," she told us.

We kept talking about Epiphany Day, when the tree would come down and we would get to eat all of the ornaments. Of course, the day after Epiphany Day, Nicola and I would have to go back to school. This gave me a very bittersweet feeling.

The next day, my father took Nicola and me to meet the landlords. When we entered their kitchen on the bottom floor, they remained seated, waiting for us to walk over to them. This behavior was a common gesture of social superiority. I had never encountered that before when living on the farm. When I shook the lady's hand, it felt cold and wrinkly. The husband's hand was warmer, but still wrinkly. We exchanged a few polite words, then left.

The structures surrounding our courtyard were one-story single rooms that were once used as barns. Now one whole family occupied each room. Like us, they had electricity, but they did not have indoor plumbing. They used chamber pots and a common bathroom.

Some of the children from the families who lived in the ground floor rooms befriended us immediately. They were so curious about how much we could or could not see that they were relentless with their questions. They wanted to know what grade we were in so they could compare notes. Once they heard us speaking they realized that our standard Italian was much better than theirs, and although we were in the same grade as some of them, we were way ahead academically.

That changed everything. Until that day the neighborhood had looked down on my family as the new peasants on the block who had just arrived from a faraway, forgotten land with blind kids away at school. The more they got to know us, the more they began to admire my family and treat all of us like humans. Now, even Maria and Biagio were accepted in the neighborhood in spite of their accent that still differentiated them from the local youth.

Biagio was seventeen, and at that point was the only one in the family with a paying job. He worked as a laborer for a local builder. Biagio worked hard to be accepted by his co-workers. He always made sure he did his work very well, and then he would help the others do theirs. My sister Maria had just turned eleven and was in fifth grade. Maria's classmates had not been cutting her any slack either. But thanks to her above-average math skills, she helped her classmates with their homework and eventually she, too, was accepted.

My mother wanted the whole family to blend in and feel part of the local culture. In spite of the insecurities she felt when around city people, she still tried very hard to always be pleasant and kind to everyone. She encountered a lot more resistance from the locals than we did, but her day finally came when she volunteered to mend something for the landlady: a garment that would have been otherwise discarded. We came from a place where exchanging services was a common daily practice, but apparently in Naples or at least in our immediate neighborhood, this was not the case. The landlady was ecstatic and very appreciative of my mother's good work—and surprised that she had been willing to do it for no compensation.

We all liked where we lived except for one major drawback. Our building was next to a cemetery. It became even more embarrassing when we had to give people our address: number 13, Cemetery Way. We often heard a horse-drawn carriage bringing a dead person for burial. Based on how many horses pulled the hearse, you could tell the social status of the deceased.

In any case, it always made me sad and afraid when they went by, no matter how many horses they had. I was afraid of death and it felt creepy to live so close to a cemetery. Only my three-year-old brother Pietro was oblivious to that fact. Moving to Naples had given him the experience of riding on a train for the first time. So now all he wanted to do was run around the dining room table impersonating the conductor of a train and calling each stop.

One day Pietro and I were admiring the Christmas tree for the millionth time when I suddenly had a brilliant idea. I thought if I slipped my hand through the branches from under the tree where there was no layer of snow, I could possibly reach a chocolate ornament, just to feel its shape. Once I did that, though, I realized it was easier than I thought to gently undo the knot that attached the ornament to the tree.

My hunger for chocolate overtook me and the ornament was soon free from the branch and in my hand. I was in a stupor of happiness, but I immediately realized that in order to avoid getting in trouble, I needed to buy my brother's silence. I first allowed him to touch the unwrapped ornament and to lick his fingers. Then, I told him that if he didn't promise not to squeal on me, he would have to settle for just that and smelling my chocolaty breath after I ate the ornament all by myself. He fervently promised me he would not tell on me, so I shared the chocolate boot I had just retrieved. I kept the foot, which was solid chocolate, and gave him the hollow leg part. I was very proud of my achievement so I quickly scouted other small ornaments that I could perhaps snatch on another day and hopefully still remain sinless.

On another occasion, I noticed that I could easily have access to another ornament from the back of the tree. If I gently pushed aside some of the snow, I could grab a chocolate cathedral. But I realized this ornament was more conspicuous than the other and someone would surely notice if it were to disappear. So I decided to partially unwrap it until I could break a section off. Then I folded the wrapper over the missing piece as though it had never been touched. I patched over the hole that I had made in the veil of snow and I happily ate some of the cathedral's façade.

In my father's search for work, an acquaintance had introduced him to a building developer who was looking for a husband and wife team to be property managers once his new building was completed.

"If you can put down two million *lire*, I can promise you a small apartment free of charge plus a stipend for cleaning and handling the security gate. You'll be set for life," said the developer.

My father paused in disbelief. He felt as if he'd won the jackpot. He thought this would be the perfect arrangement for his family.

"How long do you think it will take before the building is ready?" he asked.

"I can't give you a date right now, but everything is ready to go."

"If that's the case," said my father, "then I would be very interested, but first I have to discuss it with my wife. I have three blind kids who are away at school most of the year so a small manager's apartment would be perfect for us. Give me a few days to think about it."

"OK," agreed the gentleman.

It was a very common arrangement at the time and poor families dreamed of finding such an opportunity. The proposal seemed to be a perfect fit for our family's financial security. My mother would have work cleaning the building and my father would take care of the security gate. However, my mother was less trusting than my father.

"It sounds good, but how do you know he's not going to steal our money?" she asked.

"Our friends the Di Salvos arranged for me to meet this guy. Don't you trust them? We'll never find anything better than this offer. There's nothing difficult about keeping a building clean or checking on the comings and goings of the tenants," he argued.

Everybody in my family was euphoric with the idea of living in a brand-new building. As the caretakers, we would get an apartment with marble floors, hot and cold running water, and even an elevator. My parents would receive a small salary and not have to pay rent. The agreement was sealed with a handshake. We would finally be proud of our street address.

On Epiphany Day, the Christmas tree finally came down. My mother told us to put the ornaments in a little basket and she would divvy them up for us. When she was done putting the tree away, she looked at the basket and said, "I thought there were more ornaments than that."

My father added, "Maybe the Epiphany lady here in the city doesn't leave gifts for children without helping herself to some kind of a reward. Or perhaps we have a little chocolate monster who lives with us."

I don't know whether I looked guilty or not, but I knew that children never got scolded on Epiphany Day no matter what their sins were, so I felt safe.

Once we were back in school we began preparing intensely for First Communion and Confirmation later that spring. The school superiors informed our parents they must choose a sponsor to be present at the event. The sponsor would be responsible for renting, borrowing, or buying the fancy long white dress for this sacrament. Before my parents even moved to Naples, they had selected a distant relative who lived not too far from the school to be my sponsor. She was reliable and would be there in case my parents had not yet been able to move to Naples.

I never looked forward to catechism lessons because they were so boring and required too much memorization and repetition. I did, however, look forward to the day of our First Communion for three reasons: we got to dress up like white angels; we would receive gifts from our sponsors; and after the Mass, we would be served a special breakfast consisting of cookies and hot chocolate. I had never tasted hot chocolate before, but based on what the older children told me, it was divine. I just couldn't wait.

One day in print-writing class, the teacher handed each of us a sheet of paper on which we were to practice composing an invitation to our sponsor for the First Communion and Confirmation. We used the Regolo slate, of course, because the sponsors were all sighted people. Once the sighted assistant declared that our work was perfect, we were allowed to write the final version on fancy invitation paper. In catechism, we learned all about cleansing the soul through confession. It was drilled into us over and over that we could not receive the Holy Communion unless our soul was free of all sins, and the only way we could achieve that was through confession. Otherwise, "Jesus would cry."

The evening before the big day, we were just coming out of the chapel after our first confession when someone called me into the visiting room. On the round table where I had once stood as a five-year-old observing electric ceiling lights for the first time in my life through tear-filled eyes, I saw my First Communion dress spread out. All the staff members were admiring it and commenting on how stunning it was, but they also said it looked like it would be too big for me.

"This dress would fit Laura just perfectly. She would look like an angel with her blue eyes and blonde hair," said one of the staff.

"Carmelina could wear Laura's dress because it is a little smaller, but of course not as nice," commented another.

I was heartbroken. I was furious! It was my dress and I wanted to wear it. But of course I had no say in the matter, so I had to accept the stupid decision the grownups had made. I was so angry now at the girl who was going to wear my dress, I hated her. Suddenly a scary feeling overwhelmed me. *Is my soul no longer pure because of what I am feeling and thinking?* Now I was in a real conflict: *what should I do? I can't go to confession again.* I prayed to God for forgiveness but I didn't know whether my prayers could replace confession. *Will the Holy Mary come and reprimand me in the middle of the night for making her son cry?*

I struggled with these kinds of guilty thoughts all night long. When morning finally came, I was relieved. We were helped into our long gowns and we slowly and carefully walked to the chapel, trying not to step on the hems of our fancy dresses. Everything felt solemn, but festive. I waited with great anticipation throughout the entire ceremony for the moment I would receive Holy Communion.

When it was finally my turn, the priest held the silver tray under my chin and the bishop next to him uttered the Latin words, "*Corpus*

Dominus." I opened my mouth wide to receive the communion wafer and made sure I didn't touch it with my teeth so I wouldn't hurt the Body of Christ. The Bishop then bestowed on me the sacrament of Confirmation, wherein he gave me a light slap on the cheek. It was such a gentle pat that I wished all the slaps from adults were like that one.

After the service we walked to the room across the courtyard that was normally used for kindergarten class. There we had breakfast consisting of cookies and hot chocolate, the most delicious breakfast I had ever had in my life! I was very joyful and thankful that my dress incident had not caused a serious discord in the high Heavens, costing me a brutal punishment.

Being among the lucky ones who had family locally, I was able to leave the campus for the rest of the day. My godmother had invited my parents to join us at her house for Sunday dinner, which Italians eat at one o'clock in the afternoon. After a short siesta following the Sunday meal, we all went for a traditional *passeggiata* (stroll) along the big avenue where all of the boutiques and cafés were located. In Italy, it is customary in most areas to go for a *passeggiata* and stop for a drink, an espresso, or an ice cream in the late afternoon, particularly on Sundays.

My godmother had given me a gold chain with a Holy Mary charm as a gift for my Communion and Confirmation. I was hoping that she would also buy me an ice cream cone, but I was sure it was too much to ask. I certainly couldn't expect my parents to do it because they never had money for frivolous spending. During our walk, we passed several cafés that sold ice cream but the adults made no indication of stopping. At some point though, my godmother turned to me and said, "Would you like an ice cream cone, Carmelina?" I couldn't believe my ears! I knew I was supposed to stand on ceremony and refuse, which I did, but I hoped with all my being that she would insist. And luckily, she insisted.

We went inside and stood in line. When the customer just before us placed her order, the vendor called out the flavors and the size of her cone. The lighting was just right, so I could see that ice cream cone pass by my face. It was so big I almost died. I knew I would not be getting anything near that size (and I was right), but promised myself that on the day I received my first paycheck as a grownup, I would buy myself an ice cream cone just like that one.

I ordered my two favorite flavors: chocolate and hazelnut, but of course I couldn't be ill-mannered and ask for a large cone. The first bite was divine, and so was the next, but it was quickly gone, and I wanted more. *I hate being poor. I hate it. I hate it!*

In the fall of 1958, I started second grade and the second grade curriculum included screening for musical talent. We were all given an opportunity to take piano lessons for a number of weeks, but after that only students who had demonstrated a natural talent for music were allowed to continue in the program. At the end of the trial period, I was one of only two students selected to continue with piano lessons.

I was extremely happy to have been chosen. I liked learning to play the piano. I had finally found something that made me happy other than being at home with my family. I looked forward to my lessons and to my practice sessions every day. However, now that I'd been chosen to continue, piano study become mandatory for me and not so much fun. Piano lessons became just as serious as the academic subjects and my teacher treated it accordingly. The heavy schedule began weighing on me as I had to forgo my precious play time to practice boring scales and other tedious finger exercises every morning.

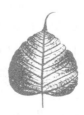

CHAPTER 44

LEARNING THE HARD WAY

Within a few months of the beginning of that school year, my brother Biagio started coming to visit us on Sundays instead of my parents. Nicola and I were happy to see him and to have a visitor but I have to confess he did not replace my mother. He usually brought us some seasonal fruits and sat mostly quiet during the whole visit. After he left, I felt even sadder than I did after my parents would leave because I would wonder why they hadn't come.

When we finally went home that summer, I noticed that my mother was less talkative than usual. She hardly spoke to us and neither did my father. It was clear that something bad was going on. We were too young to question our parents about their mood. We just tried our best not to misbehave. We waited and wondered. My father started spending more and more time at the job site where the building was supposed to be constructed. He said he was waiting for materials to arrive but they never came. Only a small pile of rebar had been delivered. Then my father would sleep night after night in a shack next to it to make sure it was not stolen.

"Don't ever grow up," my mother would say to me. "It's better to be a child and have no worries."

How could she say that? I had lots of worries! I hated being a child. That's why I wanted so much to be a grownup, so that I could be free from all of my worries and not have to go away to school anymore. I wished I could make things better for my mother, but I didn't know how.

Our landlords weren't friendly to us anymore. Whenever we walked by, they would give us dirty looks. One day I heard my mother crying in the other room while asking my father, "Where are we going to get the money to pay the rent? And how are we going to buy food?"

I knew that something really serious was up. I would learn later that the developer had taken my parents' money without a plan to ever build anything. Sometimes my mother would cry for a long time, and all we could do was wait in the other room for her to stop. Care packages started arriving from Aunt Teodora at the farm. She would send us big loaves of bread, wheels of cheese, peppers, and lard to cook with, so at least we would have something to eat that we didn't have to buy. Living in the city meant buying everything with cash every single day — something my parents were not accustomed to, having lived on their own farm for many years.

The mood was always very tense around the house. Biagio would come home every Saturday after work and hand over his entire weekly pay to my mother so she could buy food. But it was not enough to also pay the rent. The landlords would get into big arguments with my father out in the courtyard in front of the entire neighborhood.

My father's repeated attempts to get his money back from the builder failed. He would take us with him sometimes to see the builder at his house—to show that he had children to feed—but the man would not even answer the door. Naples may have been the most corrupt city in the world and so this type of fraud was a common occurrence. Unfortunately, my parents were new in town; they had been naive and trusting. My father had turned over all of his money to this man and sealed the deal with no more than a handshake. This was the only way that people made contracts in our humble community back in the high country.

Later that spring, the situation became so dire for money that my parents decided to send my 12-year-old sister to work as a live-in maid for a brief time in exchange for two meals a day. That was a turning point for my father. Unable to find any work, out of total despair he decided to take our story to the newspaper. I remember posing for the picture with my two blind brothers while my father wiped away his tears. He felt defeated. He had failed to provide for his family, and now he had to admit it to the public and accept charity. After the article was published, benefactors came to our house and brought food and money so that we could eat and pay the rent. Suddenly, every member of the landlord's family was nice to my parents again.

The Sunday that followed, my parents came to visit us at school, and in addition to the usual boring seasonal fruit, they brought candy and cookies, a previously unheard of treat for us. Plus, their spirits were uplifted. They told us all about the donations they received and how happy they were at the prospect of my father finding a job. We were ecstatic. I felt as if a burden had been lifted off my shoulders. It was a real treat to see my parents happy for a change.

In the few weeks that followed my father did receive a job offer: working the nightshift as a security guard on the docks in the port of Naples. Thanks to his experience as a war veteran, he was qualified to carry a concealed weapon. My parents were beside themselves with delight to receive this offer.

The only hurdle my father had to overcome in order to hold his job was transportation. The buses did not run late at night so he decided to buy a bicycle. Every night he would get dressed in his uniform and bike away from our courtyard into the moonlight in front of all of the neighbors who came out to watch him leave and wish him good luck. Now that my father was employed and my mother had a smile on her face again, the family became respectable neighbors. It felt a little bit like we were back on the farm.

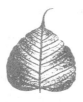

CHAPTER 45

THE BIG BANANA FEAST

One night a ship full of bananas came into the Port of Naples. Once it was unloaded, my father immediately realized that hundreds of bunches of those bananas were going to be discarded because they were too ripe to be sold. The thought of throwing away something that could be consumed by those who didn't have much food made him sick. He knew how expensive bananas were in the markets, which was why we never got to eat any at home.

He decided right then and there that in one way or another he was going to bring some bananas home. When his shift was over, he found himself a rope and strung it through as many bunches as he could and then he wrapped the whole thing around his body. Somehow he managed to drape his uniform jacket over himself, but I have no idea where he carried his concealed weapon in the middle of all those bananas. He even tied bunches of bananas onto his bicycle.

You can imagine the sight of him when he reached our courtyard that morning. He first shared with all of the neighbors and then of course with our family. It was a big banana feast. My parents even came to surprise Nicola and me at school so we could eat some bananas before they spoiled. It was so unusual for them to visit us during the week that I don't think my feet touched the ground for some time from jumping so high!

CHAPTER 46

THE SWEAR WORD

With First Communion and Confirmation behind me now, I thought the rest of my second grade year was going to be smooth sailing: my father was employed, I got to see my parents every Sunday, my grades (including my conduct) were fairly good, and I very much looked forward to my piano lessons. I did have trouble, though, observing the eat-everything-on-your-plate rule, particularly the first course which always included pasta with some kind of vegetable. Pasta with cauliflower definitely was my worst enemy.

On one Sunday afternoon after waiting all day for my parents to arrive, I was called down to the switchboard to answer a phone call. That was so unusual it scared me, but at the same time it made me feel important to be receiving a phone call. On the other end of the line was my father calling from a pay phone in a coffee bar.

He told me that he and my mother were not coming to visit me because someone in the landlady's family was deceased.

"But, don't worry, Carmelina, we will visit you next Sunday," he said.

I didn't understand what he meant by "deceased." But after we hung up, I felt hurt and outraged. *Why is the landlady more important than me? Those people don't even like us very much. All they care about is the rent money. Why are my parents helping them all the time? Damn those people!* I immediately felt guilty for using a swear word in my mind. *The next time I go to confession I'll have to tell the priest I used a swear word.*

The following Saturday evening, the priest held the routine confession before the Sunday morning communion. He sat just behind a kneeling stand, not in his usual confessional booth where he couldn't be seen. I told the priest I had said a swear word.

"You used a swear word?" he said, raising his voice. "What swear word did you use?"

I was totally confused. I had no idea how to answer.

"Which swear word did you use?" he repeated. "Why aren't you answering?" *Why is he speaking so loudly? Everybody can hear.*

I knew I couldn't repeat the swear word, especially in church or I would sin again, so how was I supposed to tell him which word I used?

"You know that the devil will come to see you in the middle of the night and he will cut off your tongue if you use swear words. Don't ever do it again!"

I could see his old, wrinkly face and his gray hair, thanks to the light that was coming in from the window across the way. His black robe was buttoned all the way up to his neck, and when he spoke I could smell his bad breath. *I wonder if the devil looks just like him? Oh no, I am sinning again. What am I going to do now?* The priest gave me a long penance of prayers—and I doubled it for thinking a bad thing about him.

For dinner that night, we were served big fava beans as a first course. They were as big as those my parents fed to the pigs when we lived on the farm. These fava beans weren't even cooked through, and in my mind they were not fit for human consumption. Of course everybody had trouble eating them, but nobody commented about them like I did.

"These fava beans are made for pigs," I said out loud. And of course, I was punished for saying that. My punishment was to stand in the corner while everybody else was getting ready for bed and to remain there until the proctor authorized me to do otherwise.

When the lights-out bell rang, the proctor forgot to end my punishment. At some point in the middle of the night I woke up on the cold, marble floor, shivering, and crying. The staff member then woke up and finally authorized me to go to bed. Later that night I awoke again. As I looked at the ceiling, I thought I saw an odd black shape floating around the night-light, even obscuring the light at times. *What is that? Am I imagining it?* I was so scared I awakened the girl next to me, hoping she could help me figure out what it was. She was totally blind with no light perception.

"Don't worry. I'm sure it's nothing. Just go back to sleep," she said.

The more I looked and looked at the black shape the closer it started circling around my bed. *Oh, no, it must be the devil. He is here to cut off my tongue.* I wrapped the covers over my head and around my body and didn't look out again until I heard the Sunday 7:00 a.m. wake-up bell. I was still in my original position, wrapped up in my covers like a log. The first thing I did was check my tongue to be sure it was still there.

Later that afternoon my parents came to visit me. I learned then the meaning of the word "deceased." The landlady's son-in-law had died suddenly of a bleeding ulcer. We had never even met the landlady's family. Nevertheless I felt badly, because the landlady's grandchildren were the same ages as me and my siblings and now they no longer had their father.

After we talked about the landlady's family for a while, my mother informed Nicola and me that we would be moving.

"Moving?" said Nicola. "Where are we going?"

"We will be moving into a room on our same floor, but at the other end of the building."

"Why?" I asked.

"With her husband gone, the landlady's daughter can no longer afford the rent on their expensive apartment, so she asked us if we would be kind enough to move to the other end of the building and to let her daughter have our apartment," she said.

"Isn't one big room with just a little kitchen too small for all of us?" I asked. "Why do we have to be kind to them? They don't even like us," I continued.

"You must be kind to people," my mother said, "even when they are not always kind to you. Now we are going to pay a little less rent and be a little more crowded, but we'll make do."

"Hopefully it won't be for too long, anyway" my father added. "Biagio is applying for a visa to go to America, so he'll be gone soon."

"America?" I shouted as I jumped out of my chair.

"Yes," he replied. "Your uncle Domenico, who's been living in New York for six years, will sponsor him."

I couldn't believe what I had just heard. "Does that mean we'll all be going to America, too?"

"Hopefully someday we will, God willing." My mother sighed. I was very happy to hear that Biagio might be leaving for America, not only because it would open up a whole new set of hopes and dreams for us, but also because it would mean I'd have one less grownup to have to answer to when I was home.

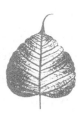

CHAPTER 47

SUMMER CAMP

At the end of second grade and again at the end of fifth grade, we had to take standardized, state-issued exams. This meant that students in those grades had to remain in school longer at the end of the school year than everyone else. The state exams were really difficult. For each subject we would first take the written portion, supervised by a teacher from a different class. Then for the orals, a panel of teachers would ask us questions at random on the various subjects we had studied during the year.

If we failed just one subject, even one as mundane as Braille drawing, we would fail the entire grade and have to repeat it. The school always offered the same exams again before the beginning of the following school year to give the students who had failed a second chance to pass the exam. Luckily, I passed all of my subjects in second grade, so I was free for the summer.

However, before we went home we were informed that Nicola and I and a few other children had been selected to attend summer camp. It was organized and offered by a school for the blind in Northern Italy, a school named for the city in which it was located—Reggio Emilia. *I've never been to Northern Italy. Everybody says great things about Northern Italy.*

The school had a site in the mountains that could house not more than thirty campers and most of the participants came from their school and ours. The school of Reggio Emilia was situated in the richest region of Italy, pretty much the opposite of our school. It had a fabulous reputation for everything: more lenient rules, the best food in the world, upscale accommodations, and everybody was happy and smiling. As interesting as it sounded, I still got a sick feeling when my parents agreed to send us there. This means one less month we get to spend at home with them, I thought. *Why are my parents always trying to get rid of us?*

"You're going to have lots of fun. It's for your own benefit. We wish we could go on vacation for a month!" they would say over and over.

In order to get to the camp, we first had to go back to school for one night on July 31. Our clothes were all marked with our usual school number and they were put in one big trunk to be shipped directly to camp so we didn't have to worry about luggage. Very early the next morning, we were driven to the train station in the school van.

Suddenly the van stopped right in the middle of traffic. At first, no one knew why the van wasn't moving. To get the van out of traffic, the staff all got out and started pushing the van full of blind kids. It was quite a sight in the middle of the chaotic traffic of Naples. The pushing didn't get us very far but provided us with a few laughs. Help did finally arrive, but we missed the train and were obliged to take a later one.

For lunch the school had packed *spaghetti frittata* wrapped in waxed paper. When it was time to eat the staffers closed the curtain of the train compartment so the other travelers wouldn't have to see what we poor, pathetic blind kids were eating. Most of the blind students who attended our school came from families of modest means, but the school could have afforded to pack sandwiches. Instead, they always seemed to choose the more miserly way out.

Once we arrived at the camp, everything seemed magnificent; even better than we had heard. We slept only five kids to a room instead of 30; the staff was sweet and kind, rather than abrupt and demanding, and the meals were way better than excellent. We were not expected to finish everything on our plates, but it was so delicious that we did clean our plates and asked for more.

Every morning after breakfast we went for a hike. We were free to climb trees, discover different types of plants and rocks, and play games. On the way back from our hike, just before lunchtime, we went straight to the water well. One of the older boys with some muscles would pump this amazingly cold and delicious water and we all took turns drinking like thirsty camels.

A long stretch of playtime followed the always-terrific lunch and then we napped. Napping was never my favorite thing because I wanted to keep moving and experience the outdoors, but it was fun to look forward to the superb snack they served afterwards: homemade bread slathered with jam that the kitchen staff made with the fruit we picked, or the same bread with my heavenly favorite, Nutella! I had never tasted Nutella before, and every time they served it my taste buds went straight into a state of ecstasy. I wondered why grownups who had some pocket money didn't buy a big jar of it and eat spoonful after spoonful until they were happy and satisfied.

The Reggio Emilia summer camp was so much fun, Nicola decided to ask the school principal, who came to visit every Sunday, if the two of us could transfer from our school in Naples to the School for the Blind in Reggio Emilia. The school principal was also blind and he had a beautiful German shepherd guide dog. When I saw the dog, I thought to myself if I'm still blind when I'm a grownup I will get a dog just like this one.

The school principal told Nicola, "I don't see why not. We would be happy to have you at our school." I was extremely excited initially, but as soon as I thought about it more carefully, I realized what it would entail: hours and hours of travel to and from the school, and months at a time without visiting with my parents. I had been through that already and I knew that no matter how much fun the school in Reggio Emilia could be, it was not worth the emotional pain that came with it.

The month at camp went by rather quickly. I had kept all the chocolate bars they had given us throughout the month so that I could share them with my family when I got home. Before we boarded the train, we each received a shopping bag containing our lunch. In it were two sandwiches with *prosciutto di Parma*, a box containing several cheeses, a box of cookies, a large chocolate bar, two apples, and a banana! No one closed the curtain on us when we ate this time, plus we could move about freely from one compartment to the other to visit other kids, boys and girls, from our group.

I saved most of the food I was given so I could take it home to share it with my family, along with the chocolate. I attended this camp for four summers in a row and every year on the trip home I was always amazed at how little effort it took to make us feel good. I wondered why our school didn't choose to treat us more like humans.

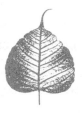

CHAPTER 48

PIETRO GOES TO SCHOOL AND I AM ISOLATED

At the start of the school year in October, 1959, it was Pietro's turn to attend for the first time. He had just turned five and was excited to go to school, just like I had been. Holding a toy truck in one hand and my mother's hand with the other he was ready to go to school, or so he thought. Nicola and I had been telling him all kinds of fun stories about school to help get him emotionally ready for the hell that was waiting for him.

He was crazy about playing the piano and could easily be distracted for hours from anything, if someone told him there was a piano he could play. In fact, that is exactly the distraction they used once we got to school so that my parents could leave without causing a crying scene. They sat him down at the piano in the kindergarten room to start the separation process. At one point my parents told him they were going to leave.

"We're going home now. We'll see you next Sunday. Are you okay?"

"I'm okay," he responded. "I'll see you next Sunday."

Between one distraction and another, he made it through the day. But at bedtime, holy hell broke loose. His dorm room was just above mine and I heard him screaming and crying with the staff member for a good part of the night. At some point they thought it would help if I sat next to his bed until he fell asleep. But he would have none of it. He wanted his mother and no one else! I wanted my mother, too, but we couldn't have her.

He spent the next week asking every person he ran into, young and old, whether they had a car and if they could take him home. Pietro's first year in school was short lived because he soon came down with a serious case of jaundice. My parents were contacted by telegram and they immediately came to pick him up and took him to the hospital. Once there, he was put into an isolation unit where visitors were not allowed. My father wouldn't hear of it. He explained to the nun in charge, "My son is sick and is also blind. He needs his mother."

"We can't make exceptions. We are dealing with a serious disease here." she brusquely replied.

"You can make exceptions! My son is only five years old and he's already traumatized from being in a boarding school. I understand, but I'm begging you, please, let his mother be with him," my father implored.

"No! She can't go in there," the nun continued.

"Well then, I'll go and be with him myself!"

"No you won't"

"Yes, I will"

"You will do no such thing!"

"What are you going to do, kill me?"

"You will go to Hell for speaking to me like that!" the nun shouted.

"I'd rather go to Hell than go to Heaven and be with a rag-head like you!" my father shouted back.

By now an Italian-style crowd had formed around the shouting match; some favoring the nun, but most on my father's side. The hospital supervisor got involved. Eventually my mother was allowed to go to my brother and stay by his side for the sixteen days he remained at the hospital. She found him lying in a fetal position, screaming with grief and shivering with cold. It took her a long time to calm him down and warm him up.

After the hospital ordeal, Pietro stayed home until our Christmas holidays. When it was time to go back to school after Epiphany Day, my parents decided that Pietro was just too young and fragile to return to school, so they kept him home for the rest of the year. That infuriated me. I didn't want to go back to school either; I wanted to be sick, too.

However, much to my dismay the day to go back to school had come, and away Nicola and I went.

Soon after our parents left us at the school, a staff member asked me to follow her. She led me into a dorm room that had only a few beds and didn't seem to be used by anyone. She told me to sit in a chair by the bed closest to the door and to wait there. I had no idea what this was about. It was mid-morning and classes were already in session.

I waited and waited in my chair for a long time, but no one ever came for me. I could hear the bells ring at the end of every hour, and that was how I was able to follow my friends' whereabouts. I wished I could be with them. I had never imagined the day I would actually be so miserable that I would prefer being in class rather than where I actually was. I tried to remember if I had done anything that was worthy of this type of punishment, but I was at a complete loss.

At one point, the door opened and a staff member put a tray of food on the bed and from faraway said, "Lunch." She then left closing the door behind her. It must have been a Wednesday, because lunch consisted of green leafy minestrone-type soup and cold cod fish salad with lemon and olive oil for the main course.

Tears started streaming down my face. I didn't want to be alone. I could taste the salty tears on my lips when I took a bite of my food. I tried to eat and not to leave anything behind because I was afraid of what might happen to me if I did.

On other occasions, when I felt sad right after my parents left, at least I had my friends to talk to and that helped me feel a little better. Now, I had no one. Between trips into my imaginary world and crying spells, the day passed. Someone came to deliver a dinner tray and pick up the one from lunch, then left quickly without saying a word to me. *What is going on? Why am I being punished? Why are people not speaking to me?*

When I heard the lights-out bell ring, I got into the bed next to my chair and somehow made it through the night. The next day, I got up with the bell and went about the morning routine as usual. Before breakfast, a staff member came into the room and said, "Come with me. You can go and join the other children now." I never thought I could experience such joy over being allowed to do what I normally hated doing.

I was never told why I had been isolated that way. Nicola told me later that he had not experienced the same isolation process. Perhaps they had to verify that I had not been exposed to a contagious disease. But why would they not have explained that to me?

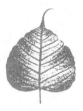

CHAPTER 49

UNACCEPTABLE BEHAVIOR

I was eager to see 1960 go by quickly because everybody at school kept saying that in 1960 the world was going to end. All sorts of theories kept floating around as to why, and it kept me in a constant state of fear. I was also becoming irritable and snappy due to what I thought were unjust and cruel punishments we had to endure at the School for the Blind. I was in third grade now and thought I deserved a little more respect.

My teacher had noticed that I was often daydreaming, therefore mentally absent from the classroom. I liked daydreaming all the time because it was the only escape I had from the constant emotional pain I experienced. In my daydreams I would leave school and go wherever I wanted and I was always a grownup and free. In my imaginary world there were no punishments and no rules that didn't make sense. Above all, I would have food, toys, and clothes that I could never have in my real life.

In an attempt to keep me engaged in the classroom, my teacher decided to have me stand next to her during the entire four hours of class each day. She would often tap my hand in the middle of a sentence and ask, "What did I just say?" She was not generous with compliments but I could tell she was impressed with my abilities in math and science, and I felt that she cared about me. I remember on certain days she would give me a Braille history book to study for hours while she worked with the other students, because they were so far behind in math while I was behind in history.

I enjoyed having this time off, but I felt trapped spending so much time indoors and sitting still. I wished she had given me permission to play outside instead. I felt fidgety and bored all the time. I wished we could have spent all day doing math, science, music, and gym. Then I wouldn't have been so miserable.

My piano teacher was nice at times, but we made fun of her because she was a bit roly-poly. She sometimes hit us over the head with a hardcover Braille music book whenever she would catch us jazzing up classical music. We were not allowed to play anything except what she assigned us, because according to her it would interfere with the development of any natural talent for classical piano.

I was one of only two students chosen to stay in her grade-school music program. This put a big dent in my playtime every morning, shortening it from forty-five minutes to fifteen, because I had piano practice for half an hour every day. I often wished I would break a finger or an arm so I could get out of practicing for a while. I couldn't believe I was actually beginning to hate playing the piano, when I had loved it so much in the beginning.

For me at school trouble was brewing. One evening after dinner, on the way up the stairs to the dorm room, Miss Malvina gave us the order to halt and let another group pass. While waiting to receive the go-ahead, some kids started talking. I was not one of them. Miss Malvina, who was looking elsewhere, turned around and shouted, "Quiet girls! Cantisani, stop talking. You're always the instigator in breaking the rules!" She proceeded to slap my face.

Before I could take a breath or think, my fist was bouncing off her chest. *How dare she slap me!* Now I've done it, I thought. I'd done the unthinkable; I'd hit a staff member and severe, unheard-of punishments would be coming my way.

"How dare you? How dare you?" she repeated with her teeth clenched. She yanked me out of the line, walked me up to the landing of our dorm room and slammed me into a corner facing the wall.

"You stay there, and don't move until I tell you. And it could very well be until tomorrow." She left me there screaming and crying.

I immediately turned around to face everyone who was walking by me. My offense was worthy of a whole new class of punishment, so whatever I did from now on didn't matter much, considering what

I had coming. A new feeling came over me then. I now felt in control.

The following morning I was awake way before the bell. When it finally rang I got ready just like every other morning, but no one would talk to me. At breakfast, I refused to eat. I might as well enjoy all the privileges that come with being a very bad child and for doing the unforgivable, I thought. This was not a matter that could be handled by immediate supervisors, so Miss Antonacci was called down from her quarters. When she arrived in the dining hall you could have heard a pin drop if not for the clickety-clack of her high heels coming toward me.

"Stand up and come with me, Cantisani," she ordered. I did not move.

"You're going to spend the day in the boys' building facing a column all day, every day, for as long as I say. You will even eat your meals standing up in their dining room," she barked.

I still didn't move. It felt really good to disobey. On the third order, I threw my chair back and stood up. My gesture angered her even more.

"Don't shrug your shoulders at me, young lady," she admonished.

She grabbed me by my left hand and dragged me out of the room and through the long kitchen that connected the two buildings. I cried and screamed. I was so furious and things were happening so fast some of the details escape me, but I do remember this: the taste and feel of her leathery, smoke-smelling hand as I chomped down on it.

The next thing I remember is standing next to a marble column crying, while all the older boys walked past me. Some of the boys even stopped to ask me what I had done to deserve this punishment. I stood next to the column all day. I ate my meals standing up at a table by myself in the boys' dining hall.

As much as I wanted to disobey and not eat, the food was actually much better than what they served on the girls' side, so I did eat some of it. Plus, they had polite waiters and no one insisted that I finish everything, so I liked this punishment. The staff soon realized that forcing me to stand in the boys' wing wasn't having the humiliating effect on me that it was meant to have. So the next day I received orders to resume my boring schedule as usual.

My third grade teacher was happy to see me back in class, but she had a warning for me.

"If your behavior doesn't improve you could very well be expelled from school. You could end up without an education and without a job, and find yourself on the street with a tin cup begging for your meals. You do not want that."

I hated being lectured to, no matter who it came from. I was so angry I couldn't speak. I wanted to tell her all they had to do was treat me with fairness and I would behave.

At lunchtime Miss Antonacci approached my table and said, "Just because you're back on the regular schedule, it doesn't mean that we are done with you. For now, no recreation time until further notice."

And so I spent all of my free time standing in a corner facing the wall. I felt like a prisoner and that I was punished unjustly. *I have to find a way to run away from here.*

The following Sunday when I was called down to the visiting room, I heard Miss Antonacci talking to my mother. She left as I approached. My mother grabbed me by my hair and sat me down in the chair next to her.

"I have enough problems to deal with at home. I don't want to come here and listen to complaints about your despicable behavior. Do you hear me? If you don't cut it out, I'll never come to see you again."

Except for reprimands, she hardly spoke to me for the rest of the visit. When she rose to leave, I stood up as well and walked alongside her all the way to the outside gate, hoping that she would talk to me. At the end of the path she strode through the gate without saying goodbye.

On the way back to the building I sat down on a stone bench with tears streaming down my face. The warm spring breeze gently lifted my hair from my forehead and the sun's rays embraced me and consoled my heart. The birds' chirping sounded friendly and I inhaled the intoxicating scent of flowers in bloom. The jasmine trees lining both sides of the driveway reached out to each other overhead, forming a cathedral ceiling. In my sad state, I asked myself: how in the world can such a lovely setting be the entryway to such a hellish existence?

I had accumulated so many punishments by then that I spent the entire week that followed without any free-time privileges. Plus, every night before bedtime I was forced to spend at least an hour standing at the foot of my bed.

One evening during mandatory study hall, while practicing our Braille drawings of the usual vase, dog, or flower, my friend Angela, often my partner in crime, and I decided to deviate from our assignment. We began to draw a person. A particular person. The feet were long, the legs and arms very skinny with an awkward body, ugly deformed head, and big hands sprouting at least eleven fingers apiece. On the bottom of my page I wrote, "school director." Next to that drawing, I drew a similar picture and wrote, "school principal."

At one point a staff member, Miss Gemma, announced it was 6:30, time for me to go to my piano lesson. Less than twenty minutes into my lesson came a knock on the door. It was Miss Gemma, with my drawings in her hands. She asked my piano teacher if she could talk to me for a moment.

"Who were you trying to ridicule with these drawings? We will see you about this immediately after your lesson," she said.

I tried to get through my piano lesson somehow, but I was very distraught and fearful trying to guess what kind of new punishment awaited me. Oh, they slapped me with a severe punishment, all right: they took away my visitation rights with my parents for one month. That punishment made me feel as if my world had ended.

That evening, I refused to eat. *There is nothing they can do to me now that is more painful than denying me the chance to see my parents.* After Miss Gemma repeatedly ordered me to eat, she decided to take matters into her own hands. She held my nose shut thinking it would automatically make me open my mouth to breathe, and then she would shove food into my mouth. But she was wrong. Instead, I clenched my teeth and managed to breathe anyway.

I won that particular battle, but they won the war that coming Sunday. There are no words to describe the pain I felt knowing that at some point during that day my parents were at the school visiting my brother, and I didn't get to see them. I knew there were three more Sundays without visitation ahead of me. I decided this pain was too great and that maybe it would be better if I became quiet and passive like some of the other children so that my visitation rights would never be taken away from me again.

On the second Sunday, my group was scheduled for a two-hour outing in the morning with Miss Malvina. Of course, still being under punishment I wasn't allowed to go. I was left in the care of another staff member with a different group. At one point the phone rang in the study hall and the staff member called out my name to go to the visiting room. I knew I wasn't supposed to visit with my parents, but once they called my name there was no way I was going to object.

Maybe my punishment had been lifted, unbeknownst to me. Or maybe the staff member didn't know and I could just get away with visiting my parents and nobody would ever find out. Whatever the case, I went down to the visiting room and found my parents waiting for me there.

During the first twenty minutes of the visit, we talked about my unacceptable behavior. I tried explaining to them I was being mistreated and that the school exaggerated my bad behavior. My parents both said to me, "Your teachers don't make up stories. If you're being punished, it must mean you were misbehaving!"

A few minutes later, my group back from their outing, started filing through the visiting room with Miss Malvina at the end of the line. *Oh, no* ... When she saw me with my parents she lost her composure. Without ever acknowledging my parents' presence, she grabbed me with both hands and pulled me away from them.

"What are you doing here? You know you are not supposed to see your parents! You know you have four Sundays without visits! Like always you are breaking the rules!"

At the sight of that, my father exploded like lightning. He jumped out of his chair, grabbed the woman by the shoulders, looked her in the eyes, and began shouting.

"Get your hands off my daughter at once or I'll kill you. When I'm with my children, if you need to talk to them, you go through me first. This type of punishment doesn't teach children anything and you're also punishing us by denying visitation."

Within seconds all of the other parents stood up and began supporting my father's position.

"This is not the way to set an example, taking the children's side in front of them," said Miss Malvina.

Pandemonium erupted in the visiting room. The switchboard operator called Miss Antonacci from her quarters to help settle the matter. When she arrived, she went through the visiting room and straight to her office, signaling to my father to follow her. First she showed my father the bite marks I had left on her hand to justify the harsh punishments I had received.

But then to resolve this heated interaction peacefully, she told my father, "I'm willing to cancel the punishments, but your daughter needs to apologize for what she did and promise never to do it again."

My father came back into the visiting room and sat down by me.

"Carmelina, you must settle down and behave like the other kids. You are in third grade now. You have to grow up. You need to apologize to Miss Antonacci for what you did. Otherwise we won't be able to see you for the rest of the month."

I hated ultimatums, and I hated even more to give in especially when I knew I was right, but I loved that my father had stood up for me. I got up from my chair and he took my hand and we walked to the director's office adjacent to the visiting room.

"Miss Antonacci, Carmelina is here to apologize to you."

I went to Miss Antonacci and shyly said, "I'm very sorry for what I did, Madame Director. I promise to be good and behave in the future."

Miss Antonacci patted me on the left shoulder and I was finally free to go and start over with a new, clean slate.

I had every intention of keeping my promise to behave, to do my schoolwork, and not be a disappointment to anyone. But the following Tuesday evening, while waiting in line for another disappointing dinner, I overheard Miss Malvina talking to another staff member.

"I have a twenty-year education under my belt. I shouldn't have to tolerate an uneducated peasant talking to me like that." That was poison to my ears; she was talking about my father. *How dare she insult my father!*

That night in bed I started planning to run away from school. I decided that the next time we were outside playing I would wander off toward the entry gate. Once I was out, I would run as fast as I could to the bus stop. I had come to the end of my rope. No more school for me. I don't care if I end up in the streets as a blind beggar with a tin cup, I thought. I wanted to go home and never come back to this school again. My head was buzzing with these thoughts of escape, bringing me some hope and comfort.

The next day, I woke up feeling good because I knew I didn't have to comply with these awful rules for much longer. At lunchtime I refused to eat, so Miss Malvina told me to remain at the table until I finished my food. Fine, I thought. I can remain here for as long as they want. Sitting here or sitting elsewhere, it is just the same to me. I will gladly skip the afternoon classes. By 3:30 p.m., I heard a clickety-clack coming down the stairs. It was my piano teacher—my classmates had told her where I was.

"Carmelina, what are you doing here? Why are you not in class?" she asked.

"Miss Malvina told me to stay here until I finish eating," I said.

"Lunch was a long time ago. Why aren't you finished?" she

asked, leaning over me and pressing her thick, dry fingers on my head.

"Because I don't want to eat. I want to run away from school and become a beggar," I said. She called over a server and told her to remove my food and tell everyone I had eaten it. This surprised me. Maybe there are some people here who care about me after all, I thought.

At the end of that school year my parents received a letter from the school stating that I would need a note from a psychiatrist certifying that I was healthy enough to come back to school the following year. I was ecstatic! Certainly the doctor would tell my parents I was sick and that I couldn't go back to school.

One day my mother told me to put on my Sunday dress and get ready to go see the psychiatrist. After we entered his office the doctor asked me to sit across from him. He left my mother standing. He started asking me questions and immediately my mother tried to answer for me. He stopped her and asked her to leave the room then swiveled his chair to face me again. Light streamed through the window on my right, so I could see his face when he spoke. He had dark hair, big eyes, and a beautiful friendly voice. He continued to ask me questions and occasionally he would write something in his notebook.

"How old are you?" he asked.

"I'm nine."

"Do you like school?"

"No!"

"Do you have a favorite subject?"

"Math."

"You're smart," he replied. "What toy do you like to play with?"

"The piano."

"You're not just smart, you're brilliant."

I could feel my cheeks pulling toward my ears in a big smile. Finally I felt happy. I would come to see him now instead of going to school and being miserable. At one point after a few more questions, he took his stethoscope and listened to my heart, then my lungs. He checked my ears, nose, throat, and at last he flashed a bright light in my eyes. He called my mother in, gave her a sheet of paper to take to the school at the beginning of the school year, and told her that everything was fine.

"Other than her tonsils being inflamed a little bit, there is absolutely nothing wrong with her," the psychiatrist told my mother.

Oh no, I thought; don't tell me I'm not sick! A feeling of panic overwhelmed me.

"You're not going to give her any medication to calm her down?" asked my mother.

"She doesn't need any medication," he replied.

"Why is she so snappy and disagreeable?" continued my mother.

"Because she is too smart and I can't treat that," said the doctor. Oh no, I thought, that means I'll have to go back to school and summer camp. My moment of happiness had been short-lived. We left his office and I was very sad all over again.

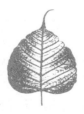

CHAPTER 50

NICOLA'S TOENAIL SURGERY

My behavior problem was not the only challenge my parents had to deal with during the summer of 1960. Nicola, now twelve, had had surgery more than once to correct his ingrown toenails, but the condition persisted. My parents were referred to a doctor who told them Nicola needed to be operated on without anesthesia so as to better kill the nerve; otherwise, the problem would not go away. Nicola was eager to have the surgery done because ingrown toenails kept him from playing soccer in our courtyard with the neighborhood kids. He was trying to be a big boy about it.

"How much can it hurt? I can stand it."

My parents were not so sure.

We kept teasing him. "Right—it's not going to hurt. You're going to cry anyway, even if it doesn't hurt!"

"No I won't," he would reply, "you'll see." After tossing the idea back and forth for some time, my parents were finally convinced by the doctor it was the right thing to do.

On the day of the appointment, Nicola got ready to go. He put on clean clothes and his usual shoes with the upper part cut off to make room for his bandages. Before leaving my parents gave the rest of us the usual sermon.

"Behave. Don't get into fights. We will be back soon; it shouldn't take more than an hour."

At the doctor's office, they tied Nicola's legs firmly to the operating table so he couldn't move them. My parents were allowed to be in the room with him. They were standing on either side of my brother, ready to comfort him because they were sure it was going to hurt quite a bit. The doctor removed the old bandages and started the procedure. As soon as he touched Nicola's toes with his surgical scissors, my brother's screams could have pierced through the ceiling. All the blood my father had seen spilled during WWII had not prepared him for this. He stepped toward the window to get some air and fainted.

My mother stayed with Nicola, told the doctor to stop and ordered the nurse to help my father out of the room. Once again my mother was trying to do her very best when things were at their very worst. She wished she had never agreed to this but the surgery had already started so it had to be finished.

When the nurse returned the doctor proceeded with the operation. Nicola was in so much pain that his screams alarmed the entire neighborhood. All my mother could do was hug him and keep reassuring him it was almost over.

My parents had not been properly prepared for the aftermath of such a brutal experience. They both felt weak and wobbly and Nicola was nearly unconscious from all the pain. By the time the ordeal was over it was way past the lunch hour, and the doctor's office staff never offered any assistance to help them get home.

My parents set off with my father carrying my brother. My mother could see that my father was way too distraught and she knew they needed to get home as quickly as possible. Their only option was to hitchhike.

Once they reached a major street my mother started waving her handkerchief at the on-coming traffic, a universal sign of distress. She hoped someone would stop and give them a ride. Finally a kind soul did stop, drove them home, and even refused to accept any money.

When we children saw our parents and brother arrive home in a strange vehicle hours after they had left, we knew that it was not good. My parents slowly made their way up the stairs and into the house.

My father gently laid Nicola on the bed and both my parents wiped away tears. I walked over to see my brother. I touched his forehead. It was hot and sweaty. He lay there mostly listless, occasionally breaking into an involuntary spell of sobs. Then he would go quiet again.

As if that weren't bad enough, Nicola's ingrown toenail problem did not go away. He had been a victim of a sadistic charlatan. A year later, he was admitted to a hospital and under total anesthesia, his problem was finally corrected. The surgeon removed the roots of the nails of both big toes completely and they never grew back.

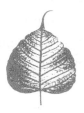

CHAPTER 51

MY EDUCATION CONTINUES

When we all returned to school in the fall of 1961, we were pleasantly surprised to find the school had gotten a makeover. The chipped paint along the staircases had been covered with a slab of travertine. The old dining tables and benches had been replaced by colorful Formica tables and slick-looking chairs. The lighting was brighter and the classrooms featured new desks and bookshelves.

"Everything feels so smooth and smells so new," said my friend and classmate Angela, "but it's still the same old prison."

Angela was one of my best friends and often my partner in crime—and she was punished at least as often as I was. Luckily, no adults heard her comments; otherwise, she would have spent several days standing in a corner during free time. But she was right. Nothing else had changed much. The food was still as disgusting as ever and everyone still barked orders at us without restraint.

Besides the makeover, the school also changed some of their practices toward the younger children. They seemed to spend more time playing outdoors and they were no longer served the usual drop of wine with their Sunday meal. Instead they received two thin bars of chocolate. I could have died with envy when I heard about that. I would have gladly traded my disgusting wine for some chocolate, but for us older kids that wasn't an option.

The younger children's dining room was adjacent to ours and we older students always had to file through there before and after each meal. My little brother Pietro was in first grade now. He sat at one of the outer tables closest to the exit, so I could say hello to him every time I walked by. As we were filing out of the dining room on the first "chocolate Sunday," I said my usual, "*Ciao*, Pietro," as we were about to pass his table. Almost immediately, he stretched out his right arm toward me to hand me his chocolate bars.

I felt total disbelief. He looked so adorable sitting at his low table. I could see well enough to discern the white cloth napkin tied around his neck, standing out against his dark blue smock. What a nice little brother I have, I thought. I could never share my chocolate with others, let alone hand it over to them. They would have to kill me first.

I should have stood on ceremony and insisted that he keep the chocolate bars, or at least one of them; after all, he was a little boy, four years younger than me, and I'm sure he liked chocolate just as much as I did. However, my ferocious appetite for chocolate got the best of me, and I accepted both bars.

"Oh look at that; so kind. The younger brother gives away his chocolate to his older sister," said his group proctor, Miss Colomba, to one of her colleagues.

That was not enough to discourage me from keeping the candy for myself. *Am I selfish for taking his chocolate? Is this something I should talk to the priest about during confession?* I quickly abandoned that thought and reminded myself that our parents would be along later and they would bring Pietro bananas, which I wouldn't get. After my brother had come down with jaundice when he first started school, my mother heard an old wives' tale that bananas helped strengthen the liver. So she made sure, no matter the cost, that Pietro ate a banana a day for years and years to come.

Unbeknownst to me, things with my family were changing quickly in an unexpected way. My oldest brother Biagio had just learned that he had the right to an American Green Card if he applied before the age of 21. This was based on our mother having been born in America and having U.S. citizenship. Biagio jumped at the opportunity and began to make inquires. Coincidently, he was due to be drafted for a two-year mandatory service in the Italian army, so as far as he was concerned, going to America was definitely an excellent option.

For my mother, Biagio's leaving was bittersweet. On one hand, she hated to see her son go; on the other hand, she thought that maybe, just maybe, this would be her ticket back to her beloved America. My mother had been only four years old when my grandfather repatriated the family to Italy. But she was old enough to remember that she always wanted to return to her beloved native land.

Her oldest sister, Giacinta (Jenny) was the only sibling who returned to New York immediately after the rest of the family moved back to Italy in 1921. By the mid-1950s my mother's youngest brothers, Dominico and Fedele, had also repatriated to America. For my mother it had not been as easy. Due to a bureaucratic misunderstanding, my mother thought she had lost her American citizenship by voting in Italy.

In April of 1961, my brother Biagio left for America. We all went to see him off at the airport.

"In five years I will be able to turn my Green Card into citizenship, and if by then the rest of the family is not able to join me in America, I will return to Italy," Biagio said.

We all hugged and kissed him goodbye. When it was my mother's turn, she broke down and cried.

"Please don't forget us," my mother said.

They both wept. My mother knew all too well that many emigrants left for America and never returned to their families.

When the plane took off my mother waved and waved, and kept repeating, "God will protect you, my wonderful son."

My mother's words made me think—possibly for the first time—about how Biagio had been the backbone of the family during the most trying times, even keeping us from starving to death when there was no money at all.

A few weeks later, my family received the first letter from Biagio. He reassured my mother that he had been well fed on board the airplane, but unfortunately when he went through customs he had to give up all the goodies she had packed for him, including the homemade salami from our home town in Basilicata.

Fifth grade was going to be particularly difficult because at the end of that school year, we had to pass the state-issued exams in order to move on to middle school, and those exams were brutal. At that time in Italy, there were two types of middle schools one could attend based on the student's grades throughout elementary school. One prepared you for a nonacademic profession of some sort. These included training to become a massage therapist or a telephone switchboard operator, the two most common forms of employment for blind people in Italy at that time. The other would prepare you for academic high school and eventual university studies to become a teacher or professor.

A fairly unusual option was a ten-year music program that my brother Nicola had enrolled in a year prior. The ten-year course of study included general education and attendance at the Conservatory of Music in Naples. It was an intensive program reserved only for music students who had the necessary talent and discipline. Upon completion Nicola would have a degree that would allow him to teach and perform. He had also moved to the adjacent building that housed all the boys past grade school and was used for all middle school classes and music lessons. Once I finished grade school I would be attending middle school classes in that building as well.

I was beginning to grow somewhat fond of my music teacher now that she had stopped smacking me over the head with a hardcover Braille music book. I was earning high grades in piano and music theory. There was hardly anything she could put in front of me that I could not handle. She enjoyed challenging me with tricky *solfeggio* sequences and complicated piano pieces.

Learning to play a classical piece on the piano was a long and tedious process. It required reading the music with one hand while playing with the other. For example, I would have to read the music for the right hand using my left hand on the Braille page. Once I memorized the notes for the right hand, I would switch the Braille reading hand and memorize the music for the left hand. Finally, I could play the piece from memory using both hands.

The teacher now trusted me with the key to her beloved classroom where the best piano in the entire school was located. She gave me permission to use it any time I wanted. She also insisted I follow in my brother's footsteps and choose music as a career.

However, I had my heart set on the Academic Middle School. In order to attend that school, you needed to have good grades throughout the elementary school years. My grades had not always been the best, but I had never failed anything. I resented their trying to choose my future for me at such an early age.

I had been with the same classmates since first grade and with the same teacher since third grade. Now in fifth grade, I still stood next to the teacher by her desk on the platform. The only exception was when she dictated notes and then I sat at my desk like everybody else. The year progressed without too many notable incidents. It helped that I had a teacher who seemed to care about me and a piano teacher whom I no longer feared.

In fifth grade our program included world history up until World War II and the tactile map of the entire globe. I especially loved the four dots on the East Coast of the United States: Boston, New York, Philadelphia, and Washington. When I touched the city of New York with my right index finger, I felt as if I were visiting my relatives and dropping in on my brother, Biagio. In my mind I just wandered around their houses and tried to imagine what their lives were like. I had heard that everybody in America had a car, a job, and more money than we had.

"I have a brother who lives in New York," I said proudly.

"You are very lucky," said the teacher.

"Maybe someday you will go live there, too, and forget all about us," said my friend, Angela.

"No, I will never forget any of you," I insisted.

As much as I hated being in school, it was going to be difficult saying goodbye to Miss Ferrara when I moved on to middle school. Teaching for her was more than a job. It was a real passion, and she cared for her students as if they were her own children.

For science projects, she would take us to the playground area where there were grasses, plants, flowers, and trees. She would have us feel and explore everything from the ground up and talk in detail about each species we discovered. She would describe to us what the sky looked like, even though she couldn't see it herself; birds flying and clouds drifting with the wind.

For me, we didn't spend nearly enough time outside exploring. Most of our classes were taught using lectures, as if we were adults. Miss Ferrara was an exception. Those lessons outdoors in the schoolyard still bring back fond memories.

"Look at this dandelion. Feel the petals and the stem."

She brought in oysters.

"You must learn everything. What you feel and what other people see. You must grow up knowing what the world looks like, not just your little blind bubble. You must become a well educated, independent adult who just happens to be blind," she would repeat over and over.

For sure, she was the quintessential example of what she preached. We all became so fond of her that we often talked about how different and difficult our lives were going to be in middle school without her love, guidance, and high expectations. We would have to tackle new subjects like algebra and a foreign language with new teachers who might not care about us.

In spite of these potential difficulties, there were definite perks associated with middle school that we were looking forward to. In middle school, some of our texts were only available in print, so sighted students from the local university would come in to act as readers in private reading rooms. This gave us a tiny bit of access to the outside world that we all craved; and boy did some students take advantage of it!

The readers were not aware of all the school's strict rules, so they were gracious enough to buy whatever the blind students requested, including cigarettes. Something that a school staff member would never agree to purchase for a student. It was in one of the private reading rooms where a girl accidentally set herself on fire one afternoon.

Like other children, as we got older we tried to engage in activities that made us feel and look like grownups. One such activity was smoking, prohibited as it was. One afternoon while the sighted reader took a bathroom break, a seventh grader named Carolina lit a cigarette that was meant to be shared by her group. After a few minutes of passing the cigarette around, one of the girls with some residual vision saw flames shooting up around Carolina's head. The girl stood up shouting, "Carolina, Carolina …" and then she fell back into her chair unable to continue speaking.

Carolina, feeling the heat from the flames, ran out of the room hoping to reach the bathroom quickly to find water. She made a right turn, and another immediate right turn, passing the music room, then to the stairway landing, and then to the left into another corridor with classrooms.

In the meantime, the sighted reader who was just coming back from her break, screamed, then fainted at the sight of Carolina engulfed in flames. Luckily, an older staff member who was drawn to the scene by the screams ran into a dorm room, grabbed a blanket and threw it over Carolina to suffocate the fire. The staff member heroically brushed flames away from her hair and removed some of the burning clothing from her body. While all this was happening, the staff member was shouting, "Call an ambulance, call an ambulance, call an ambulance!!"

The grade-school classes were already on the terrace enjoying their 4:30 break. My friend Angela, often my partner in crime, quipped, "It smells like our dinner is going to be burned beyond recognition tonight."

"Wow, that's true, but it's a really strong smell," I said.

She and I then approached the railing that looked over the courtyard. We both had enough residual vision to see the ambulance pull in.

"Oh my God!" we both screamed.

Suddenly we realized something was terribly wrong.

"Children! Under no circumstances may you leave this area! I will be back immediately," shouted our proctor as she left the terrace in a panic to find out what was happening.

When the proctor came back, she seemed dazed and could hardly speak. She seemed very different from the adult who was always in control. She asked the two oldest girls in high school to look after the younger group and left the room again. Everybody was speculating as to what was going on.

The older girls were eager to play proctor. "Stay calm. Just keep playing," they would say.

As time passed, other proctors with groups of children joined us on the terrace. Initially the staff members were very guarded. They didn't know how much information to give us. However, there was so much commotion that within a short time the entire story came out. A student had accidentally set herself on fire. Three people had been rushed to the hospital: Carolina, her classmate who had residual vision, and the sighted reader.

We spent the next several days trying to recover from this traumatic experience. Everyone seemed to be in a daze. Nothing seemed normal anymore. Finally a psychologist came to the school to talk with the students who had witnessed the accident and to help the sighted reader return to work.

Weeks later, Carolina's classmate who, due to shock had lost the ability to speak, came back. She still couldn't say complete words, only one syllable at a time. It took her at least another two months of therapy to regain her full speech. As for Carolina, she did not come back until the following school year.

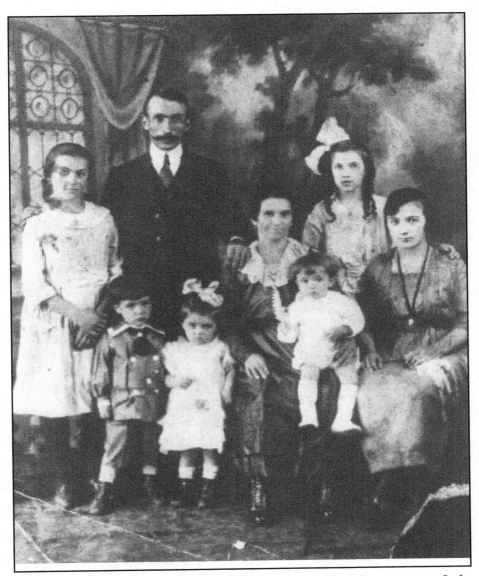

Maternal grandparents and their children the year before their return to Italy. Top, from left to right: Maria (second daughter), Pietro (father), Petronilla (mother), Feluccia (third daughter), Giacinta (Jenny, first daughter). Bottom, from left to right: Fedele (Freddy, first son), Rosa (fourth daughter), Nicola (second son).

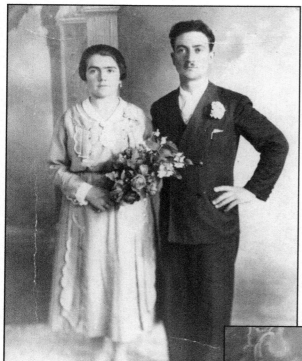

Carmela's parents' wedding picture in 1939.

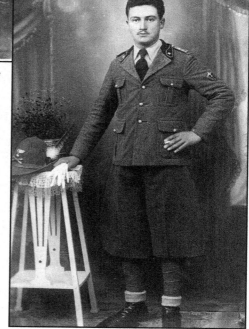

Carmela's father in his army uniform during World War II.

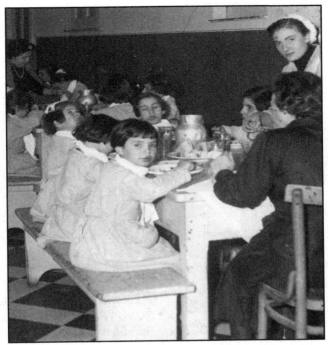

In the school refectory, Carmela looking at the camera.

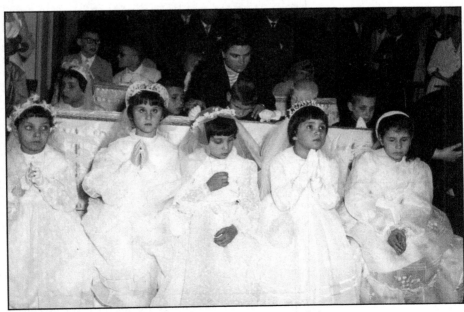

Carmela at First Communion (second from the right).

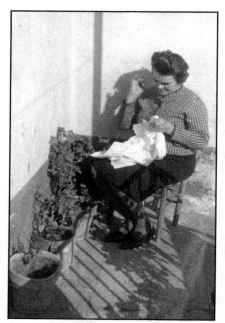

Carmela's mother in front of the one-room apartment in Naples.

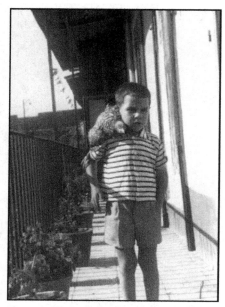

Pietro (Peter) with a chick on his shoulder in Naples.

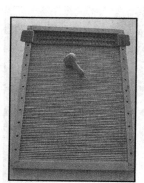

Braille slate Carmela used in first grade to learn how to write and to emboss shapes.

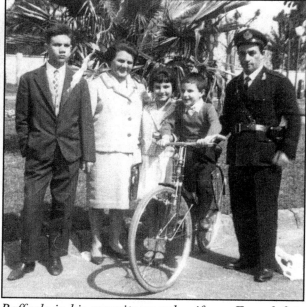

Raffaele in his security guard uniform. From left to right: Nicola, Rosa, Carmela, Pietro, and Raffaele.

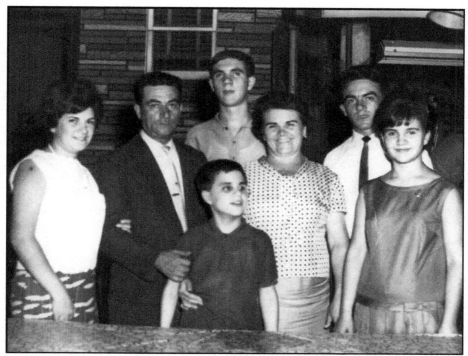

Carmela's family reunited. Photo taken one week after their arrival in New York, in August, 1964. From left to right: Maria, Father, Nic, Mother, Benny (Biagio), Carmela, and Peter in front.

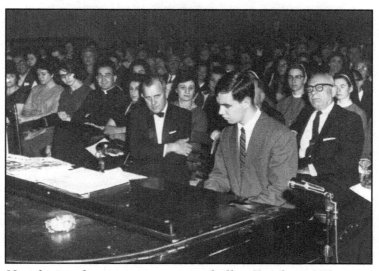

Nic playing the piano in a concert hall in Younkers, NY.

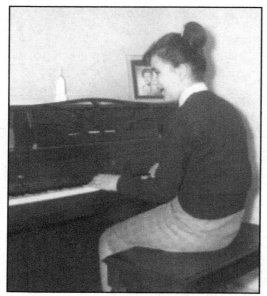

Carmela playing piano as a teenager.

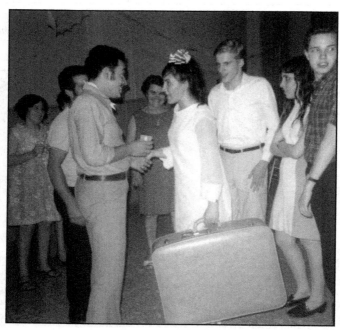

Carmela receiving new luggage before going away to college.

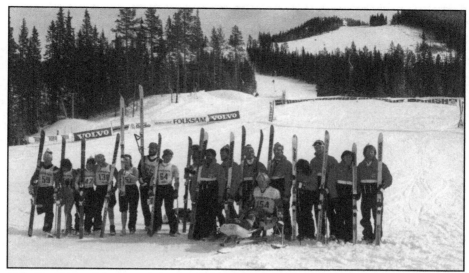

US Ski Team for the Disabled, 1986 World Championship in Salen, Sweden (Cliff and Carmela, 1st and 2nd on the right).

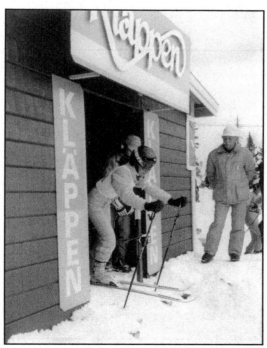

Carmela at the starting gate of the downhill race, 1986 World Championship in Salen, Sweden.

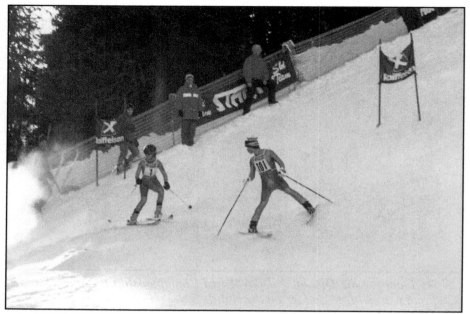

Carmela and ski guide Cliff in the downhill, 1986 World Championship in Salen, Sweden.

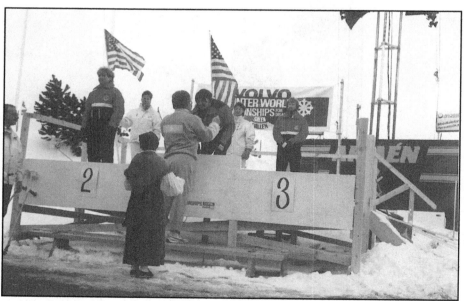

Carmela receiving a gold medal, 1986 World Championship in Salen, Sweden.

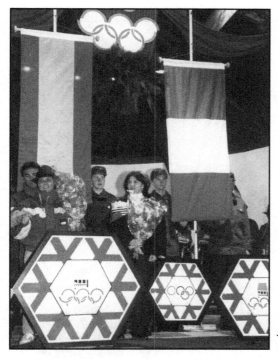

Carmela receiving a bronze medal, 1988 Winter Olympics for the Disabled in Innsbruck, Austria.

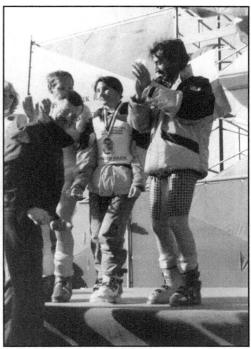

Carmela receiving a bronze medal, 1990 World Championship for the Disabled, Winter Park, Colorado.

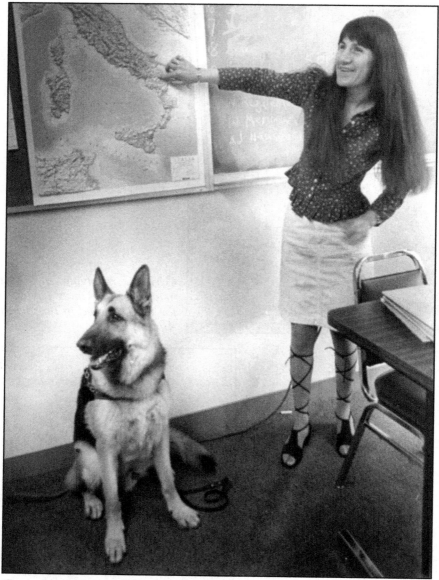

Carmela teaching Italian at the Defense Language Institute indicating her place of origin, the Basilicata region in Southern Italy. At her side was guide-dog McCloud.

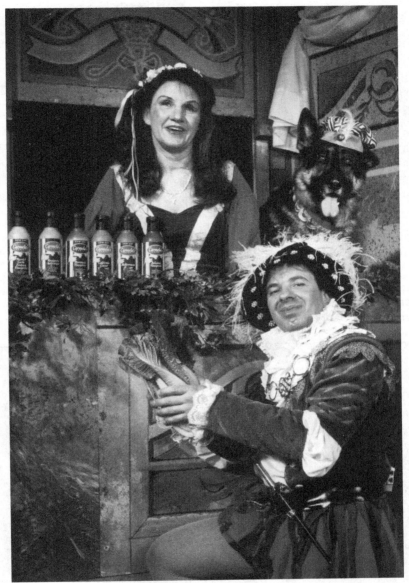

Among their many adventures, Carmela and her husband Gilbert, turned their passion for cooking into a Specialty Food business that grew and lasted for a number of years. This photo was part of Carmela's Gourmet display booth featuring her line of gourmet salad dressings. Gilbert and Carmela posing as Romeo and Juliet with guide-dog Heinz.

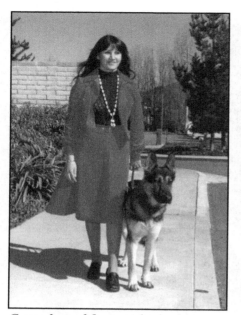

Carmela and first guide-dog Colton.

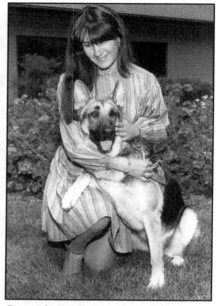

Carmela and second guide-dog McCloud.

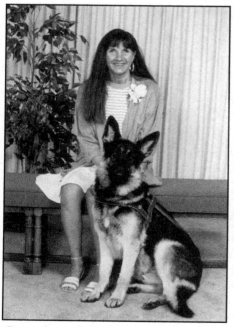

Carmela and third guide-dog Heinz.

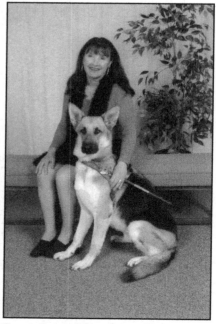

Carmela and fourth guide-dog Loomis.

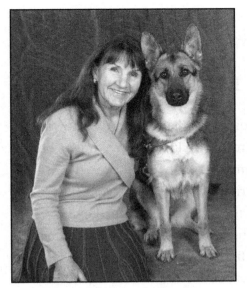

Carmela and fifth guide-dog Luna.

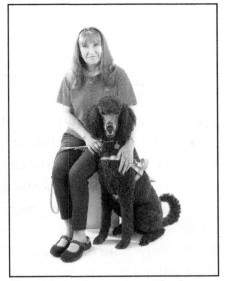

Carmela and current guide-dog Seymour.

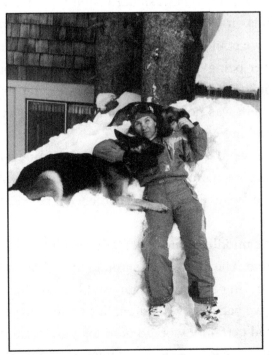

Carmela on the snow with the only two guide-dogs that overlapped, retired Heinz and young Loomis.

CHAPTER 52

SLEEPING ON THE BATHROOM FLOOR

As spring sprang forward, loquats and cherries started showing up for dessert at the end of each meal. We knew it was time to buckle down and start reviewing and committing to memory every word from our notebooks we had diligently written with a Braille hand slate.

Traditionally, students preparing for the state-issued exam would get up early to study every morning, well before the wake-up bell. It was the only extra time we could find in our busy schedules. None of us owned a watch, so we had to set our internal clocks and hope they would work. The bathroom was the only place we could gather to study as a group. Those with some residual vision would check the window for any sign of dawn. If it still looked pitch black and we were finished with our work, we could go back to bed until the bell rang.

I remember being so sleepy during this time. The studying was grueling and sometimes one of us would fall asleep on the cold bathroom floor because there was no choice. Nobody wanted to risk repeating a grade just for making one small mistake.

The exams were very involved. The academic portion consisted of essays, poetry recitation, and clear and accurate answers to oral questions. There were no multiple choice or True/False versions to make it easier.

Around the middle of June, all students not taking the state-issued exams went home. The atmosphere around the school was calmer then; but between worrying about the exams and looking forward to the long summer break, we had plenty of adrenaline to keep us going. We all felt prepared. We had certainly worked hard enough, or so it seemed to us. Even in knitting we had achieved our goal: we could do several fancy stitches and knit the four pieces of a pullover sweater. And for the art portion of the exam, I had worked all year to perfect embossing a *fleur-de-lis*, free-hand, on a Ballu slate.

First on the schedule were the written portions of the exams, which included free-hand embossing of an object. The desks were spaced far apart to make sure no one could cheat. The doors connecting the classrooms stayed open and numerous proctors and teachers circulated.

By the third day it was time for the orals. I remember walking into the classroom for the history and geography test. The room was full of teachers sitting at their desks with writing material in front of them. My teacher, Miss Ferrara, stood in the front of the room next to a table that held a tactile map of Europe and next to the table stood the tactile globe that we had been studying the entire year.

When I walked up to her, she gave me a very warm, kind greeting. She took both of my hands in one of hers and gave the globe a spin. When it stopped spinning, she put my right hand down on it and asked me to identify and talk a little about what I was touching. I immediately recognized Mount Everest. I began talking about the Himalayas.

"*Bravissima*!" she exploded. She was proud of my performance and I assumed she was equally happy to show off her hard work in front of the other teachers. She held my hands tight and gave the globe another spin. This time we landed in Chile, the long, skinny country with a mountain range running in the middle of it from top to bottom that always reminded me of the spine of a fish. She asked me some questions about its population, the names of major cities, and its industry.

Our final stop was in Europe. She asked me a number of questions that combined history and geography, more detailed than before. I was able to answer each question correctly. When she was done, she asked the panel if they had any questions for me. They all declined.

"Very good," they said. I floated out of that room on cloud nine. I knew I had done well and that I had passed.

The only exam left now was the oral in music. I had already taken the performance portion of the test. I had answered the questions and played what I was asked to play, but without much passion or interest. I hoped I would receive a low grade disqualifying me for the music program.

Within a week all of the exams were over and we said goodbye for the summer. As far as I was concerned, I was ready to begin the Academic Middle School in the fall.

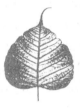

CHAPTER 53

A LOVE/HATE RELATIONSHIP WITH MUSIC

When classes resumed in the fall of 1962, I discovered that instead of being enrolled in the Academic Middle School like I wanted, school officials had enrolled me in the music program. I protested and asked to be switched.

"The Academic Program is closed already," they told me. "You should be grateful that you have the talent. Not everyone is so lucky. And you should take advantage of it."

A surge of rage came over me. I couldn't believe they could decide my future without consulting me! I was very disappointed and angry.

Being in the music program did have some advantages. I would have a lot more freedom, much more than any of the students in other disciplines. But I would also spend a lot of time studying and practicing by myself. All that solitary time would be too difficult for me. I knew deep down that I had succeeded in grade school chiefly because of my support system: my classmates, who were of course my best friends, and my excellent teacher.

The teachers in the music department would ask my brother Nicola to come see me every day to try to convince me to remain in the music program. While he was with me, I felt the confidence necessary to continue with music. After all, in spite of my mean grade school piano teacher, I still loved music and I was good at it. But, as soon as he would leave, I immediately would start reliving the nightmare I had experienced in grade school with my piano teacher.

When she was in a good mood she would say, "You are very lucky to be musically talented, but you have to build strong hand muscles while you are young; and only play what I give you or you will ruin your development of a good technique." I don't remember her ever giving me a compliment.

When she was in a bad mood she made sure I noticed every single mistake I made. Once when I was playing a popular song and didn't think anyone could hear me, she came running into the practice room, grabbed a hard-cover Braille music book off of her desk and hit me over the head with it. "I told you not to play that garbage. You can ONLY play the music that I give you!"

I started hating piano lessons so much that sometimes I would go as far as hurting my own fingers in order to avoid playing. I came away from that experience with a love/hate relationship with music that I have never been able to resolve.

With the exception of one or two students, my old classmates were all enrolled in the non-academic middle school. Whenever we saw each other, they would say, "We really miss you. We wish you were with us. Things aren't the same without you." This warmed my heart.

It was clear to me then that I needed their companionship and support if I wanted to enjoy any form of happiness in the hostile school environment. The system had betrayed me and I would have none of it. So, I officially removed my name from the music program and enrolled in the non-academic middle school. At least there I was in the company of good friends.

In middle school our living arrangements changed. We now slept in a smaller dorm room with only eighteen or nineteen beds instead of thirty. We had a dressing area where we each shared a wardrobe with another girl. In it we kept our classroom uniform: a black smock with a white, snap-on collar. It was the national uniform worn by all Italian students attending public schools. I liked my black smock uniform. I finally felt like a legitimate student, instead of a blind prisoner dressed in a pathetic blue-and-white checkered smock. It was exactly in this dressing area that one could still see a black spot on the floor where the girl engulfed in flames had been saved by a staff member a year ago.

Every morning after breakfast we would spend at least 20 minutes doing stretching and orientation exercises before class. We had been doing these exercises since first grade. I had thought we wouldn't have to continue doing them in middle school, but I was wrong. After stretching, we would march in formation for several minutes.

When the proctor gave the command to disperse we would continue marching in tempo, but in whichever direction we chose. "Disperse! One. Two. One. Two. Keep moving! One. Two. One. Two. Knees up, no shuffling! One. Two. One. Two. Keep changing direction! One. Two. One. Two. No bumping or touching! One. Two. One. Two. Heads up, shoulders back, keep moving! One. Two. One Two. Back in formation! One. Two. One. Two. No touching, no talking! One. Two. One. Two."

When the proctor gave the "Back in Formation" command we had to continue keeping in step while we tried to return to our original position. We weren't allowed to talk or touch each other in order to benefit fully from this exercise. The proctor's voice was the only point of reference we had to orient ourselves. However, we did find a way to cheat just a little. We each had our own secret grunting code to help us get back in place.

The purpose of this exercise was to develop spatial vision. It is the ability to identify the presence of solid objects by hearing the contrast between empty space and full space. Our senses had to be on full alert to make this work. This is how we learned to move about gracefully and with self-confidence. While we lived at the school, we were never introduced to the concept of using a white cane, because we were expected to put our orientation skills to work at all times.

Once we were finished with these exercises, we would file into the adjacent building where middle school classes were held. This building had been added to the main structure the year I was in kindergarten. In fact, it had been during the early stages of its construction when I had sadly dropped and lost Tomasina's beautiful harmonica. It was also where all the boys lived once they were out of grade school. Our classes, though, continued to be segregated. The school maintained a strict divide between the sexes as we approached puberty, so just the thought of being in the boys' building stirred up unfamiliar emotions in the girls.

Our middle school was also a district middle school, so at least half of the students were sighted. But like in elementary school, all the teachers were blind, with the exception of the typing and P.E. teachers. This was a great way for the School for the Blind to integrate us into the public school system.

For us, it was a huge deal. We looked forward to being in class, side-by-side with sighted students from the outside world. Because the school was located in an upscale area of the city, most of the sighted girls were day students from affluent families. Unlike the blind boarding students who came from all over Southern Italy, many from poor families.

It felt good to meet new people, even though at times we felt awkward, unsure of ourselves, and insecure about whether we were up-to-date with the world. The ambiance in middle school was definitely different. Everything seemed unfamiliar and scary.

One by one, we met all of our teachers. I knew immediately that I hated my math and science teacher. And for sure, I detested my French teacher. I wanted to be a grownup so badly, I couldn't understand why someone who was already an adult would squander such a privilege by being so dry, unfriendly, and unfashionably dressed.

The other teachers were acceptable, but it was clear that not one of them was going to look out for my sensitive self like Miss Ferrara did in elementary school. I was on my own now and I was scared. Miss Ferrara knew how easily I could slip away into my daydreams to avoid the unpleasantness of the present and worked diligently to keep my attention so that I could succeed in all my subjects. Now, the only classes I looked forward to were typing, weaving, and P.E. because in those classes, I didn't have to apply myself mentally, and thus I could daydream all I wanted.

CHAPTER 54

LEARNING ABOUT THE COMPLEXITY OF LOVE

In New York, my brother Biagio had been diligently facilitating all the steps necessary for my father to immigrate to the United States. In the fall of 1962, my father was cleared for immigration, and he began preparing for his departure in March of 1963. Now a sense of excitement filled the air. The prospect of all of us moving to the United States in the foreseeable future suddenly became more real.

Daydreams about my family enjoying a lifestyle possible only with a higher income had been hopelessly looping around in my head for as long as I could remember. Now I had a feeling dancing in my heart, that my daydream could take shape in real life. This was the topic of conversation during every Sunday visit with my parents before Christmas break.

It was hard for me to imagine, though, what life was going to be like at home without my father. Would my mother and my sister be scared living by themselves? Who would stick up for me in school if I got in trouble? Nevertheless, the idea of moving to America and finally leaving the awful School for the Blind was intoxicating.

In his letters to my parents, Biagio had been mentioning that he had met a special young woman by the name of Michelina Di Gennaro who was crazy about him. She hoped with all her might that Biagio's family would emigrate to New York. Michelina had immigrated to the United States from the region of Abruzzi at the age of eight along with her parents and her older brother. Her family lived in the close-knit Italian American neighborhood on Beech Street.

While Nicola, Pietro, and I continued our studies at the School for the Blind, Maria had perfected her trade as a custom shirt-maker and had already secured a position with the highly regarded Ricci seamstress in

Naples. She got dressed up and took the bus downtown each morning. She really enjoyed working with other girls her age.

Their boss, Mrs. Ricci, was an extremely meticulous and very energetic eighty-year-old. To make sure her employees did their work with precision, she did not allow them to talk except for the recitation of the rosary every afternoon. Maria would often tell us about the discreet laughing fits she and her coworkers would have as they were reciting the rosary. They had found a way to insert quick words within the prayers in order to exchange "boy gossip."

"Hold it right there girls," Mrs. Ricci would say when a customer entered the shop. While she was waiting on the customer, Maria and her friends would whisper and laugh.

She inevitably forgot where they had left off, so upon her return one of the girls would resume reciting the rosary very close to the beginning so they could continue to gossip while praying.

With his departure imminent, my father grew concerned about Maria's commute to downtown Naples.

"Not everyone's intentions are honorable," he would say, "especially if they get wind that the man of the house is absent."

My parents decided to purchase a commercial-grade sewing machine for Maria so she could start building a clientele of her own at home. They felt this would be a safer way for her to continue working once my father left for America.

Initially, my sister was not in favor of this decision. She enjoyed the routine of getting out of the house and going to work in one of the most elegant areas of downtown Naples. But eventually she embraced the idea of having her own clientele and setting her own prices instead of working for someone else. Mrs. Ricci was disappointed to lose a good employee, but was so impressed by Maria's skills that she sent some of her own clients to my sister.

When my brothers and I got home for Christmas that year, my sister's work area with her new sewing machine was already in place and through word of mouth, she was starting to build an impressive clientele. The wonderful smell of new fabric permeated the air. I was excited. I thought for sure she was going to have pieces of leftover material every now and then and that maybe she would use it to sew something for me. Just the idea of wearing something new, made just for me, gave me butterflies.

My first morning home, I got up, washed, had breakfast, and proceeded to tackle the list of chores my mother had asked me to do for the day. I enjoyed giving her a break; plus, as the one in charge of cleaning, I got to push my brothers around with some legitimate authority.

While my mother did the daily food shopping, my father slept, because he still worked nights as a security guard. Maria labored at her sewing machine; and Nicola, unable to practice the piano with my father sleeping, entertained Pietro by playing games with him.

As I dusted the furniture, it seemed I could hear my mother's words in my head: whether you are rich or poor, live in a castle or a shack, if the place is dirty, then the inhabitants are pigs. The house had to be spick-and-span from top to bottom before noon every day as though we were expecting the Queen of England to join us for lunch.

So I cleaned. Before sweeping and mopping the floor, I made the beds and dusted the furniture. After doing the armoire, I decided to do what I always did on my first day home. I went through my sister's clothes, which were stored in the armoire. I was curious to see if she had gotten anything new. Eventually, I knew I could expect to be wearing it in the future. When I started feeling through her things, I could not believe what my fingers were telling me ... There wasn't just one new item in her closet or just one new outfit. There were two new, outstanding ensembles with a new pair of high-heel patent-leather shoes with a decorative design and a matching purse.

I was livid with anger and jealousy. I nearly dropped to the floor. How could this be possible? I asked myself. How could they do this to me? I sat on the bed I had just made. I could hardly breathe I was so angry. How could they be so insensitive toward me? Didn't it matter to them that since the age of five, I had been miserably sad at school, away from home, dressed in a school uniform, wearing underclothes and scuffed-up Mary Janes that had been worn by other children? And didn't they care that when I came home, I had always worn my sister's hand-me-down clothes that never fit me right? Did they not think about me at all when they went shopping for all of these beautiful things?

Was it possible they just didn't have one *lira* remaining that they could have spent on a lousy piece of leftover material to make me a dress? Did they just not care about me at all? Both my mother and my sister knew how to sew! I sat on my bed with my head down and clenched my teeth; I listened to my heart pounding in my chest for a long time. I wasn't going to let them get away with this.

When my mother came back from her shopping, she didn't notice me right away. The curtains separating the sleep area were drawn. She went straight into the kitchen to put the groceries away. When she came into the big room to inspect my work, she asked, "What has gotten into you? Why are you sitting on the bed during the day doing nothing? Why the angry face?"

I didn't even look at her. She got closer and closer to me and kept asking the same thing. I didn't answer. She finally noticed the armoire door was open and immediately determined the problem.

"I see, you looked at your sister's clothes, didn't you? Your sister is a young lady now. She is working and she needs to look presentable. Doesn't that matter to you? Is that a good reason to stop doing your chores? If I'd stopped in my tracks every time things didn't work out for me, you would have all starved to death a long time ago."

I did not care one bit what she said. I remained immobile. I was too hurt to do anything else. I hated her and I hated everybody.

"Get rid of your anger and make it fast or I'll give you something legitimate to be angry about!" she said as she went back into the kitchen to fix lunch.

By then my father was awake and about the house. He asked me what the commotion was all about. I didn't answer. There was sort of an unwritten rule in our family that when one of our parents was on fire with one of us, the other one would try to put it out. This time I had set the fire and I had no plans to put it out. When my mother came in to serve lunch, she ordered me to sit at the table. I didn't move.

"What seems to be the problem?" asked my father.

"She is mad because her sister got some new clothes," said my mother with an angry tone.

"And for a new dress, you're making all of this fuss? Why didn't you just say you wanted a new dress," asked my father.

That question made me even angrier. I didn't know I had to remind you to love me, I thought. I hated everyone and everything. I wanted to run away. Why was it taking so long for me to become a grown-up? I decided right then and there I was going to take the easiest and the shortest route to a paying job so that I could leave home and never come back.

They ate lunch without me, realizing it was best to leave me alone so they could eat in peace. I heard my mother say, "When she gets hungry enough, she'll eat." Whenever I heard her say that, I would think to myself, "No, I'm never going to eat again until things change."

After the cleanup from lunch, my sister went back to the sewing machine and my mother came to sit across from me.

"What are we supposed to do? Grant your every wish? You snap your fingers and you should get what you want? Don't you know that you're still growing and we can't afford to buy clothes that you're only going to wear once or twice?"

Oh, don't play poor with me; I don't want to hear it. I continued to ignore her. Realizing that her words were having no effect on me, she became overcome with anger and frustration. She yanked me off the bed by my right arm and slapped me a few times.

"I told you I was going to give you a real reason to cry!" she shouted.

I pushed her away with my left arm and she nearly fell backward.

"You are a disgrace to my life!" she growled through clenched teeth. "How dare you! Only someone as evil as you would have the nerve to hit her own mother!"

My mother sat down at the dining room table, holding her head between her hands. This was an indication it was time for her to vent. Whenever my siblings and I engaged in ugly behavior she always blamed it on our paternal genes, but this time she didn't dare because my father was present. My temper tantrum had triggered her memories of every misfortune in her life, and right at this moment, of course, it was all my fault.

Now for hours we had to listen to her long litany of ways she had been short-changed in life. All the sacrifices and all the tears she had shed. In her mind it had all gone unnoticed. I have been crying for years too, I wanted to tell her, but unlike you, I have been doing it without an audience. At that moment, all I wanted to do was lash out and hurt everyone the same way they had hurt me.

At dinner everyone ate quietly. I remained sitting on my bed.

The next morning I got up, washed, got dressed, made my bed, and resumed the same position as the day before. My father had already come back from work and had gone to sleep. When my mother went out to do her food shopping, my sister went along with her. They did not dare to ask me to be their Cinderella that morning, because they knew that I would ignore them.

Once they returned, Maria immediately went back to work. My mother remained in the kitchen. After a while, she came into the large room and walked toward me. When she was about three feet away from me, she stretched out her right arm and held a tube of rolled-up new fabric under my nose.

Oh yes, my face lit up, but the joy was bittersweet. *Why do I have to go through such agony every time just to get a smidgen of what I deserve? Why do they seem to care so little about me? Why are they so blind to what seems to me so obvious?* No matter how many such questions I asked myself over and over, I could never come up with a satisfactory answer.

"Go stand next to your sister so that she can measure you," my mother said firmly, holding back tears. I had been stewing in my pain and anger for more than twenty-four hours. It would take me a while to simmer down.

On Christmas Day, I set the table and put the customary Christmas letter we all wrote to our parents under my father's plate. The letter was written in Braille, double-spaced, and under each Braille line I had printed the same words with the Regolo slate. After dinner, my father read it out loud. I wished them a beautiful, holy Christmas, and a prosperous New Year. I also promised them I would behave and work hard at school. Afterward, both my parents expressed their gratitude, complimented me on my nice writing, and gave me a 50 *lira* coin.

Unlike in previous years, this time I had an unsettling feeling about the letter. *How truthful was the letter? Will I be able to keep the promises I had made? Was I lying? Was I guilty of a sin? How did this work?* It didn't make much sense to me then; but years later I realized I had just had my first taste of the complexity of love in the real world.

My new dress was ready for me on New Year's Eve, my twelfth birthday. We had been invited by our landlady to watch television with her, her three children, and other neighbors until midnight. It was the only television in the neighborhood. I didn't like watching TV much, because I just couldn't see the screen well enough to discern what was going on.

But I didn't need entertainment anyway because I had my new dress. I was ecstatic. I couldn't stop touching its beige wool with fine threads of different colors. The dress had long sleeves, was fitted at the waist, and had double pleats down to my knees. With some strips of leftover material my mother had made roses, which she had sewn onto every other pleat just a few centimeters above the hemline with a button in the center that matched the buttons on my sleeves and on my chest.

I couldn't believe what a good job she had done. She was so talented! I felt pretty enough to be scooped up by a charming prince and ride in a silver carriage, just like the ending of Cinderella. I got to wear my beautiful dress again the next day for the beginning of the new year and then it was put away until the next winter holiday.

My father's departure date for America was approaching quickly. So once we were back to school after Epiphany Day on January 6, 1963, my father made a trip to our hometown in Basilicata to say goodbye to the family. I thought about him visiting our relatives. It had been so long since we had left the farm that I wished I could have been with him instead of back in school.

My paternal grandfather had died years and years ago, but my grandmother Mattia was still alive and in her early eighties. She lived with her daughter, Antonia, my father's youngest sibling. My father always stayed with them on those rare occasions when he was able to pay them a visit. This visit was emotionally charged, with long and tearful embraces day after day as he made his rounds to all his siblings, their families, and all the relatives and friends he had known his whole life.

I can just imagine how painful the final goodbye to his mother must have been for him. My grandmother was old and frail. My father knew he would never see his mother again. This was the dark side of emigration. As a child I could scream my pain when I said goodbye to my parents, but how do adults live through it? Was it as painful for them as it had been for me?

When the time came for my father to leave his mother they simply embraced and wept together. Tears and silence best replace words when the pain is too hard to endure. When my father was finally able to let go of her, he turned around and slowly walked away.

CHAPTER 55

MY FATHER LEAVES FOR AMERICA

One mid-morning in March, a knock came on my classroom door. Once the teacher gave the go-ahead, my group proctor stepped inside after coming from the adjacent building.

"Mister Cantisani is here to say goodbye to his daughter. He is leaving for America tomorrow."

"Go ahead, Carmelina," said my teacher, "You can leave the room." I had been expecting this day for some time, but didn't think it would affect me the way it did now that it was here. My emotions were scattered in all directions. The word "America" sounded so real, so far away, so exciting; but what if this was the last time I would ever see my father? What if the ship sank? What if it took years before we could join him in America? I knew he would never forget about us—nevertheless, at least a million what-ifs rushed through my head.

I stood up, passed the window on my right and the two rows of desks in front of my own, turned left, went by the teacher's large, elevated desk on my right, and straight out the door.

"Carmelina, I came to say goodbye. I'm getting on the ship for New York tomorrow," my father said. My heart pounded. I was so overwhelmed with emotions I didn't know what to say.

"I want you to promise me you will work hard, always do your homework, and not get in trouble in school. And make sure that when you're home, you behave for your mother so she doesn't get upset. Since I'm going to be gone, things will be harder for her. If everything goes well, soon you will all come to America and we will be together again."

Although my father had been coming to visit every Sunday, it was even more special to see him in the middle of the week. Nothing ever interrupted classes except emergencies or unusual circumstances. I was so sad to see him go. He leaned over and kissed me on both cheeks and I kissed him. He smelled so good; like the outside world.

"Take care of yourself, my little one," he said. Then he put two 100 *lira* coins in my hand. "Spend it wisely," he said. "Buy yourself something good." This generous gesture shocked me out of my sadness a little bit. I had never been given this much money before that I didn't have to turn over to someone. Immediately, I saw a stream of ice cream cones parading in front of my face. I had enough to buy myself four large ice cream cones dipped in dark chocolate.

"I'll write as soon as I get to New York. I'll send you my address so that you can write to me," my father said, holding back tears.

I returned to my classroom with half of my heart weeping and the other half leaping with joy at the thought of one day going to America, as I fingered the 200 *lire* that I had slipped into my uniform pocket. I knew every one of my classmates wanted to be me at that moment. And for a change I wanted to be no one else but who I was.

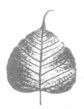

CHAPTER 56

THE LOVE LETTER

About two weeks later, I was called to the visiting room during the free-time period after lunch. I figured it was probably Nicola; maybe he had received a letter from my father. Then I realized my father hadn't been gone long enough for a letter from him to have arrived yet.

When I walked into the visiting room, there was Nicola, and he did have a letter for me, but not from our father. It was a love letter written in Braille from an older boy, Fabio, who was trying to court a girl in my section, Daniela. It needed to be delivered in secret.

The girls and the boys were so strictly separated in our school, it was nearly impossible to have any contact with each other. We rarely even shared the same space. Occasionally, we would all attend musical performances by outside artists, but even then the boys sat in the back of the room and the girls in the front.

It must have been at one of those concerts when she was sitting in the last row of the girls' section and he in the first row of the boys' section that a bee pollinated Fabio's heart with Daniela's nectar, and he fell madly in love. Or, perhaps he simply got a whiff of her pheromones and was love-stricken. Whatever the circumstances, Fabio wrote a harmless letter professing his feelings to his beloved Daniela.

Every single move we made was so scrutinized that I decided I'd better not give her the letter until after lights out that evening. The proctor would be tucked away under her tent and I would quietly tiptoe to Daniela's bed and slip her the letter. But I did tell some of my classmates about the letter. What harm could there be in that? The plan seemed fool proof. I had gotten up that morning with a bad headache that kept coming and going all day. During free time before study hall, I sat on a bench not feeling quite right.

My friend Angela came over and asked me, "Why aren't you playing with us?"

"I'm not feeling so good," I replied.

She touched my forehead and dragged me to see the proctor, Miss Gemma. She confirmed that I looked sick and took me to the infirmary. The nurse, Miss Lucia, checked my temperature and showed the results to the proctor without saying a word. They both seemed puzzled. The nurse put the thermometer under my arm again to double check my temperature. When she removed it she showed it to the proctor, and they both said, "You need to go to bed immediately." They then proceeded to put cold packs on my head.

In the meantime, my sixth-grade classmates were uncontrollably curious. As soon as study hall began, Rita and another classmate took the letter out of my book bag and started reading it. Of course it was written on fancy, shiny Braille paper and did not look like homework. As soon as Miss Gemma spotted the letter, she immediately confiscated it.

Although sighted, she knew Braille well enough to read the contents of the letter. As much as my classmates wanted to protect me, it was impossible for them to hide the truth. Within minutes the entire secret operation was exposed and Daniela, the intended recipient of the letter, identified.

The school director, Miss Antonacci, was immediately contacted. The matter was serious. She did not come onto our floor, but from her living quarters she prescribed a month of punishment for Daniela and her entire eighth-grade class of four girls. The punishment required Daniela and her classmates to stand in the four corners of the visiting room during free-time.

About three hours later while hallucinating in my bed with a high fever, I felt the nurse shake my shoulder gently.

"I have a message for you from Miss Antonacci," she whispered in my ear. "Don't worry about anything. It doesn't matter what you did. Everything is fine. Just get well."

"Doesn't matter what I did? What did I do?" I was confused, because I did not yet know that my classmate had taken the letter out of my book bag and caused holy hell to break loose.

The next morning, with a clear head, I was able to read between the lines of the director's message. It seemed that she and all the staff involved had assumed my high fever was caused by the shock of being caught with that letter. Luckily for me, that was not the case but I was grateful for the priceless coincidence which helped me escape a severe punishment. I was relieved by her assurances, but saddened when I learned that the people who were being punished were not the least bit involved in the intrigue. To our surprise, Fabio, the initiator and love-stricken young man, and the two couriers (Nicola and me) went scot-free.

A month later, when the would-be Juliet got her freedom back, she approached me during free time, all giggly and happy. "What did the letter say?" she whispered in my ear. I was surprised and relieved to see that she wasn't angry with me for causing the whole mess. In fact, she was flattered and her friends were all amused by the disproportionate punishment given for such a benign and innocent transgression.

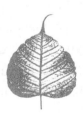

CHAPTER 57

FAILING SIXTH GRADE

Throughout this school year, I steadily fell behind. Unlike our grade school teacher, Miss Ferrara, our new teachers didn't really seem to care about us or our personal struggles. They projected a sink-or-swim attitude that did not sit well at all with me. I felt abandoned by my teachers.

I think we worked just as hard as before, but those of us who were blind were now required to read some of the material through readers because the texts were not in Braille which made it that much harder to absorb the information. By the beginning of May, it was fairly clear to me that the prospect of passing my final exams was dim. I was not alone, though. At least half of my blind classmates were in the same boat.

We had also learned that starting with the next school year, the non-academic middle school was going to be abolished. There would be only one type of middle school for everyone. I liked that idea; so it didn't bother me a bit if I had to repeat sixth grade. Attending a combined middle school made my future seem a little less confining.

As I feared, I failed most major classes, including math, which was very unlike me because it had always been my best subject. When students failed, they were given a chance to retake the exams in the fall before school started again. My parents couldn't afford a private tutor for the summer, so repeating the grade was a given.

Ever since my father had emigrated to America, our plans to join him were becoming more and more concrete. Not knowing when, exactly, we would emigrate, my mother wanted to make sure during the summer of 1963, we would spend time visiting our relatives in our hometown in Basilicata. Our finances had not allowed us to visit them since the family moved to Naples, in the fall of 1957, and this would be our last opportunity.

CHAPTER 58

DANCE PARTIES

Our new apartment was located just at the top of the outdoor staircase, only two doors down the covered walkway from where we used to live. It consisted of one large room and a long narrow kitchen. At one end a heavy curtain separated the kitchen from the toilet area. The kitchen had small windows and was equipped with an old cone-shaped sink with cold running water. In order to wash dishes, do laundry, and take baths, we had to first heat some water on the propane burner and fill a utility basin. This kitchen had been added to the main building in recent years without giving much thought to structural support.

One evening when we were watching my mother cook, she said, "Remember what your father used to say: if you all gather in the kitchen too much weight might cause the building to tumble away with all of us in it!"

"At least the cemetery is right next door. We would save on the price of the horse-drawn hearse," said Nicola.

"Stop joking about death like that!" my mother shouted. "It's a sin and it's bad luck." My brother, Nicola, was a clever fellow. He knew exactly how to push my mother's buttons to get the right reaction for our own amusement. But he was also very careful not to push his luck so far that he earned himself a slap; but if he did, he timed his get-away perfectly so my mother's slap would always land in mid-air.

With both my brother Biagio and my father gone, having less living space didn't seem to be a problem at all. Between receiving money from America, paying less rent, and my sister making money from her sewing business, our lifestyle improved significantly.

The large room where we all lived had a high ceiling and one window. It was separated into two parts by a long drape. On one side was our bedroom furniture. On the other side stood the dining room table, the piano, Maria's sewing machine, and two other pieces of furniture. Back when our family was destitute, we had received a beautiful upright piano from the Red Cross to help Nicola with his music studies. It was the only piano for miles around. Some years later he also received a reel-to-reel tape recorder from our district to assist him further.

We were all becoming gregarious teenagers. We shared the same circle of friends and they all seemed to gather at our house. Nicola was already an impressive piano player and we all enjoyed singing and dancing to popular tunes he played.

It didn't take us long to turn these gatherings into a full-blown dance party. We would simply draw the drape open, push the dining room table close to the beds, and suddenly we had a fairly good size space for dancing. And much to our benefit, we never had to worry about making too much noise because our landlady, her children, our neighbors, and their children were all part of the fun. Naturally, the residents of the cemetery next to our apartment never complained. Throughout the evening my mother would even pass around a cordial with some lady fingers. Those parties gave us the opportunity to experience our first innocent flirtations, sometimes accompanied by love at first sight.

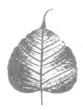

CHAPTER 59

GOODBYE TO THE FARM

As planned, we spent the later part of the summer of 1963, visiting relatives in our hometown in Basilicata, something we hadn't done since we moved to Naples. My mother decided we would stay with my father's brother, Uncle Giuseppe, and his wife Anna. Although their house was small and still had no running water, they lived in Seluci, the only town in the farm community that now had electricity and a general store within walking distance.

My siblings and I were not that excited about going back to the country. We were city teenagers now and each obsessed with our friends, contemporary music, and the latest fashions. We were not proud of our simple country roots. Spending our summer vacation stuck out in the boonies was not something that would impress our city friends when we returned home. Maria worked late every night at her sewing machine to finish all of her custom shirt orders before we left.

By the early 1960s travel to our hometown had become more convenient and took less time. Instead of multiple trains, there was now a direct bus from Naples to the nearest town of Lauria. In Lauria, my Uncle Giuseppe's brother-in-law, Vincenzo, picked us up in his van and drove us the rest of the way to my uncle's house in Seluci.

I was completely surprised by the warmth and love we received from extended family that we hadn't seen for so long. I suddenly realized that for the past seven years in Naples our friends had replaced family, but now I could feel the difference between the two. There was no holding back from my aunts, uncles, and cousins. Hugs and kisses were exchanged, and tears of joy flowed freely down every cheek. We felt loved and knew what it meant to be part of a large extended family. It felt good.

Readjusting to the old way of life took some time, particularly using the outside toilet and having to pump water from the well. However, the first bite of homemade bread took me back to my early childhood on the farm when happiness was the only feeling I knew.

I woke up the first morning on my uncle's farm to the singing of the rooster. I could see light coming through the shutters, but it must have been early because everyone else was still sleeping. We were all sleeping in the same room, but I felt the moment was mine alone. I quietly left the bedroom and tip-toed to the front door. As soon as I stepped outside my first breath of fresh country air came loaded with memories.

I walked away from the house a short distance and sat on a patch of shimmering grass that was wet with the morning dew. I realized suddenly why it felt so good to be here. This was where I spent my early childhood years when I was happy and knew nothing but happiness. Unfortunately, it all came to an abrupt end at the age of five, when I had to go away to a residential school for the blind to get an education. It was there where I learned for the first time in my life the bitter taste of real tears and perpetual, gnawing sadness.

I listened to the birds cheering on the sunrise, the gentle rustle of leaves, the sounds made by tiny creatures moving in the grass, and other whispering noises nature makes that can be heard only in the absence of cars, motor scooters, street vendors, noisy neighbors, and other man-made racket. I looked at the sky and wondered how long before I would hear the rest of the sounds of this wonderful land: the donkeys, goats, sheep, the cowbells. I felt sad that I couldn't share my feelings with my siblings, because I knew that if I admitted how much I really liked it here they would start calling me a farm girl and I'd never hear the end of it.

Once back in the house, my uncle Giuseppe and his wife Anna were up and ready to go to work in the fields.

"You're up early. Did the rooster wake you up?" asked my uncle.

"Yes," I replied. "I haven't heard the sound of a rooster since we moved to Naples."

"Well, we'll see you later on this afternoon," he said as they both left for the day.

Over breakfast, each of my siblings had something to say about the inconveniences of farm life and how backwards everything seemed and looked. I felt a pressure to join in, so over a glass of freshly drawn cow's milk and a slice of my aunt's homemade bread topped with local honey, I complained about having to go outside to use the outhouse and not having running water.

Nicola had already made more than his share of disparaging remarks, but the final blow came when he said, "I bet there are people around here who still think the earth is flat instead of round." Then, realizing the gravity of what he had just said, he pushed back his chair and made a beeline for the front door.

My mother, who was standing by the stove and already involved in preparing the midday meal, grabbed a polenta stirrer and ran after him. Realizing that she couldn't catch him, she stopped at the door and shouted, "I'll break this polenta stirrer over your back into a million pieces, you hear? This land is where you were born and these people are your family, and don't you ever forget it! If I hear any of you say something of that sort again I'll split your skull in half!" She turned back into the house, angrily throwing the polenta stirrer back into its corner.

Total silence permeated the room. Unfortunately we had pushed the wrong buttons and stirred up her frustrations and the pent up anger she had been accumulating for years. It was right here in Seluci where the Cosentinos resettled when her father repatriated the family back from America in 1921. And it was here that she had to live with all the consequences of her father's catastrophic decision. Yes, at one time she might have been one of those people who thought that the world was flat, because no one had taught her any different. If the family had stayed in America, she would have received an education and learned more about the world than just its shape.

It was also here that she gave birth to three blind children who brought her years of guilt and despair. Unfortunately, these traumas often caused her to view life as a struggle rather than an interesting journey. Actually, it was the birth of her three blind children that gave her the opportunities she wouldn't have had otherwise. Because of us, she moved to the city and learned to fit into an entirely new culture. If we hadn't been blind she might never have left the farm at all.

We knew that it was best for us not to be around her right then, so we all tip-toed out of the room as if we were walking on shattered glass. Luckily, my aunt and uncle were already out in the fields working so they didn't witness our despicable behavior.

Within a day or two, all the relatives, neighbors, and friends from near and far started coming to visit us. They brought bread, cheese, salami, corn flour for polenta, vegetables from their gardens, and live chickens and rabbits, so that we would have food for our entire stay.

One mid-morning, my mother busied herself in the kitchen preparing to kill one of the chickens we had received as a gift. I was really looking forward to dinner because in the city, we never ate chicken—not at school and not at home. It was just too expensive and the sources not altogether trustworthy.

I was standing by the door when suddenly the bird with half its neck slit open, flew by my face, splattering blood in all directions. My mother was surprised to find that she had lost some of her dexterity for such an operation. Close to death as it was, this chicken still managed to fly and squawk. I wished I could save it, but my mother was angry at the chicken for escaping and making a mess. We finally caught the bird and cleaned up the kitchen. Dinner turned out to be not only delicious, but the source of a good story.

Nicola had brought along his reel-to-reel tape recorder, not only to play music but also to record messages from every relative who came to visit us. Most of them had never seen a tape recorder before, and they were flabbergasted to encounter a machine that could repeat everything they said, word for word, and in their own voices. When word got around we had such a machine, everybody came to tape messages to the relatives in America.

We enjoyed our relatives' company and being on the farm, but as typical teenagers we were eager to get back to the city and resume our faster-moving lifestyle. But it was still painful to say goodbye for the last time to all the relatives, especially the older ones like our paternal grandmother, who for sure wasn't going to live long enough for any of us to see her ever again.

One chick remained in the coop from all the gifts we had received when we had first arrived. Uncle Giuseppe insisted we take it with us.

"No, no, no," my mother insisted, "it will be impossible to take it on the bus."

"Sure you can; this is a gift for little Pietro," said Uncle Giuseppe. Pietro continued to whine about wanting to take the chick with him, until finally my mother gave in. She put the chick in a wicker basket with a linen cloth over it, and there it stayed all the way home.

In Naples, we were delighted to have the chick. We played and played so much with it that it became a pet to us and all the other neighborhood kids. It would eat out of our hands and follow us around, especially little Pietro.

"In all the years I've been around chickens I've never seen one so affectionate," said my mother. She even took pictures of Pietro with the chick standing on his shoulder.

When it was time for us to resume regular classes in early October, it was hard to say goodbye to the chick, knowing we would have to wait until Christmas to see it again. On Sundays when my mother came to visit us, she always told us our little pet was fine. But when we arrived home for the holidays, there was no chick to be found.

"Where's the chick?" Pietro asked.

"I didn't want to tell you at school, but one day it escaped. Maybe it was caught by a hungry animal, because it never came back."

Pietro was devastated. He cried about not having his best friend anymore, but at least he believed my mother's story. I wanted to believe also, but I knew she was lying. I found out some time later that the chick had ended up in the roasting pan shortly after we had gone back to school.

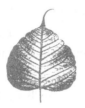

CHAPTER 60

HAIR STYLES AND HIGH HEELS

In January of 1964, a new proctor joined the staff. She was young and I thought she was really cool. Her name was Miss Carletta. She wasn't as strict and as overbearing as the other proctors. She wore her uniform for only the first two weeks on the job and then she started wearing street clothes. She wore straight skirts discreetly above her knees and her hair was stylish with blonde streaks. *Is Madame School Director letting her get away with that?* I don't know whether she got in trouble with her superiors for wearing street clothes instead of her uniform, but she certainly kept doing it. I loved her nonchalance and her beautiful, stylish shoes. I wished I could trade places with her.

Within a few weeks a new girl enrolled in school. While she was undergoing the customary initiation (a bath and final surrender to the school uniform), the staff discovered she had lice. This precipitated a scrub-down of all the students in the school.

As it was, we were already required to keep our hair short and tidy. But if one student had lice, the school immediately rushed a barber to the scene to shave every child's head. Then he applied a powder that smelled for all the world like DDT. It was torture. Our hair was our only means of declaring an identity by wearing a headband or other simple ornament like a bow or clip. Now that possibility was gone. The wait for our hair to grow back was long and painful. I felt so humiliated that as soon as my hair was long enough, I decided to rebel and do something creative with it.

One Saturday night I washed my hair with cold water and a big bar of soap in the bathroom sink. I cut two sheets of used Braille paper into three sections, rolled each section nice and tight into a tube, and used them as rollers to set my hair, anchoring them down with bobby pins.

The Braille dots worked well to help keep my hair from slipping off the homemade rollers. The next morning I combed my hair out, teased it, and styled it into a nice bouffant, knowing full well this was against the rules and would most likely earn me a punishment.

When we lined up to go downstairs for Sunday Mass, Miss Carletta did her usual check to make sure we were all groomed and dressed properly. She took me aside and hollered to the others, "Hold it there, girls!" I was sure she was going to ask me to comb out my hair and wear it in a simple style like the other girls. Instead, she took me under her tent, sat in her chair, put a comb in my hand, and said, "Do my hair like yours."

Miss Carletta? The person immediately in command over me, is willing to become my partner in crime? Does she really love what I have done to my hair that much? I was flattered and empowered. I realized at that moment I had more than just friends my own age in this school. I teased her streaked blonde hair and carefully smoothed out the surface with the comb in my right hand as I shaped it with my left hand into a bouffant style that matched mine nicely. When I was finished, she looked at herself in the mirror and said, "I love it, let's go."

Even with Miss Carletta's approval, I still had the jitters walking downstairs through the visiting room and through Miss Antonacci's office to reach the chapel. Luckily Miss Antonacci wasn't in her office.

Once inside the chapel, I figured I was safe. I didn't think anyone in that school had the nerve to yank me out of God's pew, slam me into a corner, and deny me the right to Sunday Mass with communion. After all, I could recite the entire Mass in Latin by now and there must be some divine protection in that from the high Heavens. So I prayed.

The following Saturday night, I wasn't the only girl who set her hair. Miss Carletta had bought herself a set of real rollers and a can of hairspray to finish the job. The next morning our little dorm of fifteen girls became a full-blown hair salon. I couldn't believe the fun we were having, and all it took was a young staff member who understood harmless, girlie pursuits. A year or two earlier, I would have been thrown into a cage of hungry wolves for doing something so absolutely innocent.

Now that I was in sixth grade and taking a typing class, I was eligible to apply to my county of origin, Potenza, for a typewriter. I received not just any typewriter, but a beautiful Olivetti. The first thing I typed with it was a letter to my father in New York. When I received his response only three weeks later, I was crazy with joy to have a letter from such a faraway place. I couldn't believe what I was holding in my hands.

I sniffed the letter to see if it smelled like my father. It did! When I unfolded it I held it up close to my eyes and I could see my father's writing on the page. I wished that I could see well enough to read the letter myself.

Attached to the letter I found a dollar bill. *A whole dollar bill? A whole dollar for me?* I just couldn't believe it. Oh yes, life was good. Now I really felt like a grown-up. I actually owned paper money for the first time ever. Now I could afford to buy my own can of hairspray and every day I'd look like I'd just stepped out of a beauty parlor.

On Sunday mornings now I got up way before the seven o'clock bell so that I would have enough time to style everybody's hair. And every Sunday the line at my "salon" got longer and longer. Yes, we were breaking the grooming rule, but I was doing such a professional-looking job that soon even the other proctors would get in line to have their hair teased, styled, and sprayed.

I loved visiting Miss Carletta under her tent and playing with her dozen pairs of high-heeled shoes. She seemed so normal and unthreatening compared to the other staff members. She didn't keep her shoes neatly arranged in her armoire. They were all scattered on the floor next to her bed. As luck would have it our feet were the same size. When I tried on her high heels, I felt sick with impatience to be old enough to wear such shoes.

One morning, I went to her tent to do her hair and felt the shoes she was wearing.

"Oh, they are so beautiful!" I said. Immediately she slipped them off and told me I could wear them.

"What?" I said, "I can wear your shoes?"

I looked at her in disbelief, with my heart bouncing out of my chest.

"Yes, you can wear them to class, and then take them off when you come back and change into your regular uniform."

Oh my God! I thought. What if Miss Antonacci sees me? I wondered how many years of punishment I would accrue by breaking the rule about appropriate footwear. Oh, never mind, I thought. I surrendered. I simply couldn't pass up the opportunity.

I slipped off my scuffed-up Mary Janes and on went the most beautiful, strappy, dreamy shoes. I glided like a dove. I knew exactly how to walk in high heels from years of practice with my mother's and sister's shoes in secret. But this was actually the first time I wore a pair in my size. *Would Miss Carletta get in trouble if I got caught?*

I concentrated very hard going down the stairs to make sure my body movements were no different from normal. I bent my knees a little so I didn't look taller than everyone else. The real problem was that in order to get to the adjacent building, the boys' side where the middle school classes were held, we had to walk through the visiting room—which was next to Miss Antonacci's office.

I prayed her door would be closed. When we walked through the visiting room not only was her door open, but she was standing with two other proctors watching us walk past her office. I feared the worst.

When I made it past her without being caught, I was beside myself with relief. How did this happen? Had I concentrated so hard at not being visible that I had actually become invisible? Perhaps Miss Antonacci had seen me, but just when she was about to yank me out of the line and throw me in a corner, she remembered my teeth marks on her hand from years before and then immediately envisioned one of my strappy high heels being driven through her skull.

Somehow or other I made it to the boys' building in high-heeled shoes. I felt glamorous and was one million times happy.

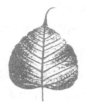

CHAPTER 61

WAITING TO IMMIGRATE

In late February of 1964, my family was called in for the final clearance to immigrate to the United States. Once at the American Consulate in downtown Naples, we were fingerprinted and told to wait in a large hall packed with other families from all over Southern Italy. While waiting for hours and hours, we met all kinds of people hoping to immigrate to various places in the United States to join loved ones. We all exchanged addresses and promised to write one another once we started our new lives on the other side of the world.

When our number was called, we were led into an office where a female agent was waiting for us. She wore a straight long skirt way below the knee, jacket to match, thick high-heeled shoes, and her hair in a tight bun. She asked us several questions in Italian with a beautiful American accent. She was sweet and very kind so we forgave her for her extremely conservative and very dated outfit. (My sister and I had no idea what fashion snobs we were.) When she informed us our date of departure was not to exceed sixty days, Nicola immediately asked if it was possible to extend the date until the end of June.

"I am in the fifth year at the Conservatory of Music and I would like to complete it so that if I return to Italy for any reason, it will be easier for me to go straight into the sixth year," he told her.

"We can postpone the date," she responded, "but that means you will all have to come back and go through the final clearance again. Is that OK?"

My mother resisted changing initially. She had been waiting for this day for so long she didn't want to risk jinxing it for any reason. Reluctantly she agreed to extend the 60 days. With much apprehension on my mother's part we then went back to the usual grind, waiting to be called again.

CHAPTER 62

THE BOYS REVOLT

The month of March was fairly uneventful, except for the long-awaited celebration of St. Joseph Day on the 19th. It was one of those rare times when the school served dessert with our meal. The traditional dessert for St. Joseph Day is "*zeppole*," consisting of a beignet-type doughnut filled with pastry cream.

We were all extra well-behaved during dinner the evening before St. Joseph's Day. We wanted to make sure our special treat would not be taken away from us. While eating quietly, a very loud noise that sounded like a huge stack of dishes crashing onto the tile floor startled us. Initially we thought the incident had happened in the long kitchen that connected to the older boys' dining hall. A few seconds later some of the proctors left their tables and hurried toward the kitchen to see what had happened. When they came back they all gathered in a group and began whispering amongst themselves.

We were dying of curiosity to learn what had occurred. Little by little the information trickled down. We heard there had been what they referred to as a "revolution" on the boys' side. Apparently a group of boys had planned to create chaos in the dining room to protest against the school rules and the food.

At dinnertime two boys had gone to the utility room and cut the electricity once everyone else was seated. As soon as darkness permeated the room a boy who had some residual vision gave a voice signal. At the signal everybody in the dining hall simultaneously stood up and flipped their tables upside down, breaking every dish, every glass, and every jug of water. They proceeded to smash the tables against the marble columns or the floor to make absolutely sure each table was broken into at least four pieces. All of the perpetrators were blind but they had carefully choreographed the entire event to be sure no one was injured.

Somehow one of the proctors made his way out of the dining room in the dark and managed to go to the switchboard and call the police. The police responded immediately and for several days we had a police presence everywhere inside the school.

Details about why the boys had rebelled were sketchy and slow to reach the girls' side of the school. But we did notice a sudden improvement in the quality and preparation of the food. We were grateful for that. To our surprise soon after, the general rules became a little bit looser.

Initially, no one was held accountable for the revolution because in the dark it was impossible for the proctors to identify who was doing what. But eventually, two boys who were eager to get expelled from the school did come forward and identify themselves as the main organizers. During the few days it took for the school to contact their parents and have them picked up, we often heard them singing popular songs with guitars in their courtyard. Perhaps they were practicing to enter the new chapter in their lives as blind beggars, playing for their meals in the dirty and chaotic streets of Naples.

I wondered what went through their minds. Were they worried? Were they scared about what lay ahead? Or perhaps they were singing because they no longer felt incarcerated like the rest of us. They were happy to be free at last.

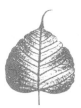

CHAPTER 63

A BURDEN TO SOCIETY

By the end of April, we were at the American Consulate again for another final immigration inspection. We met a whole new room full of people immigrating to the United States with whom we exchanged addresses as we had the first time. The second agent who interviewed us did not speak Italian and was not very friendly. We waited impatiently for her to give us the approval we had received the first time. This time it wasn't going so smoothly. She reviewed our paperwork several times and consulted a large manual on her desk. A very long pause followed.

"Why isn't she looking at us?' muttered my mother under her breath in Italian. "Something isn't right; I know it!"

Finally, the agent spoke to us through an interpreter.

"As things stand right now, in order to immigrate with three blind children you or your sponsors must deposit a $2,000 bond for each blind child. It will not be refunded to you for five years."

My stomach turned. I knew we didn't have that kind of money. My future was ruined. I would have to spend many years to come at the School for the Blind in Naples.

My mother could hardly breathe.

"Why do we have to deposit this money?" my mother asked. "My children will be going to school in America just as they are here."

"I know that," the agent replied, "but we need to have some guarantee that your blind children will not be a burden to society."

"A burden to society?" my mother asked.

"That's the law and I cannot change it," the agent said in a heartless tone of voice.

There was no way we could come up with $6,000. It is all over, my mother thought. Her lifelong dream to return to her beloved America, her wonderful land of birth, had vanished. She immediately started blaming Nicola for not keeping his mouth shut during our first interview.

"If you hadn't said anything we would be in America already by now and none of this would have happened! Now, we get to stay here and be poor forever. Are you happy? You just ruined everybody's future."

We left the consulate troubled and disappointed. The rest of the day was a nightmare. My mother, in total despair, hurried to send my father a telegram with the terrible news.

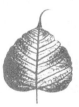

CHAPTER 64

RELATIVES TO THE RESCUE

Back at school we could no longer brag that we wouldn't be returning the following year. And when we went home for the summer, we said goodbye to our friends and the staff as though we would see each other again the following fall.

Meanwhile as soon as the news spread among our relatives in New York, they mobilized. My mother's two brothers, Domenico and Fidele, her sister Jenny, Jenny's five grown children, Great Aunt Rosina who had helped my mother raise us on the farm, and Biagio's future in-laws all chipped in as much money as they could to raise $6,000. They were determined not to stand by and accept such devastating news without putting up a big fight.

They were fully aware their money would remain unavailable for five years. Everyone in my family was a blue-collar worker, so $6,000 in 1964, was a heck of a lot of money. As soon as the $6,0000 bond was secured in the bank my father received the green light to send us five airplane tickets to America.

In early July 1964, we received five one-way airline tickets departing from the Capodichino Airport in Naples to New York. We were to fly on August 16.

Once my mother had the tickets in her hands nothing could stop her from smiling and sharing the news with anybody who would listen. She put the word out to sell our beautiful piano and arranged to have my sister's professional sewing machine shipped to America along with a trunk full of things that were dear to us. She wrote to my father's siblings in our hometown and offered them our furniture if they could manage to pick it up a day or two before we left. They were grateful for the offer and made the arrangements.

We all received new outfits for the trip. For the boys it was simple. They wore slacks and polo shirts. A professional seamstress made my mother's outfit. My sister made her own with a blue silk fabric using one of the latest styles from a fashion magazine. I designed my own dress using a stunning piece of raspberry-colored satin crepe that I had received as a going-away gift from my godparents. A professional seamstress turned my design into reality. It was a beautiful dress that still hangs in my closet today.

As soon as the word was out that we were leaving for sure, people started coming from all corners of town to record on tape their best wishes, along with poems, songs, and jokes for us to take to America as souvenirs. It was everyone's unattainable dream at the time to go to America, so we were considered extremely lucky. Some people hoped that maybe if their recorded voices made it to America, somehow one day their bodies would follow.

Although school was not in session, my mother got us all ready and took us to say goodbye to the school principal, the school director, and any staff members who happened to be on campus. As I shook everyone's hands and heard them wish us all the luck in the world, I couldn't help but notice how pathetic they looked to me now that they no longer had the power to control me.

As we were leaving the campus I savored every step I took, and thought how much sweeter this moment would have been had it happened during my earlier years at the school when life there had been the most difficult. We walked through the courtyard, then the archway, and the big open space that narrowed into the path that led to the front gate. I was blissful as we walked through it for the last time, crossed the street, and stood on the sidewalk waiting for the bus.

It was a bright, sunny day, and with the little bit of functional vision I had, every contrast I could see seemed clearly defined. I looked at the gate for the last time and could even make out the beginning of the path that had led to such a hellish existence for me for so many years.

When I finally lowered my eyes, I noticed the white lines in the middle of the street that separated the lanes and the bus stop sign on the pavement. Whenever I had walked out of the school on previous occasions, I was always floating on such a high cloud that I never noticed anything around me. But this time I was delighted to stare at every detail. After all, I was never coming back. However at the tender age of 13, I had no idea that being separated from my parents at such a young age, being punished unfairly over and over, and being forced to follow strict rules that stifled all my spontaneity would impact me for the rest of my life.

Before we left for America my mother organized a day trip with our closest friends. She wanted us to tour the attractions of the city of Naples as a family, something that had been out of our reach because we never could afford it. We visited the Amalfi Coast for the first time and several other popular sites. We rode in a horse-drawn carriage through the historical center of the city, a luxury we had only seen tourists enjoy.

I remember on many occasions being downtown on foot when the sun was very hot and bright, wishing that I could be riding in one of those carriages, and now I was. I was wearing a pair of stylish sunglasses Maria had bought for me, a blue linen skirt, and a cream silk blouse she had sewn for me. And let's not forget the black mesh and patent leather shoes and purse to match. I looked as chic as it gets! I tried not to feel guilty about all the people who had to walk in the heat as we had always done before.

We shared almost every last night in Naples with our neighbors and friends. We would spend our time reminiscing, dancing, and singing along to romantic popular ballads. Some of us would sneak out onto the long balcony hoping to share an intimate moment with a heartthrob or a secret admirer. The bright moon was always present, sitting on rooftops watching over us relentlessly like an old, nosy grandmother. It was beautiful.

We would stay up well into the night and our friends would go on and on imagining our lives in America. They teased Maria about marrying a rich American who would take her on a long honeymoon to Italy.

"You and your rich husband will come back to Italy by ship and you will disembark with a big Cadillac. It will be so long that it will cause historic traffic jams in the narrow streets of Naples."

"You are crazy," Maria would say, laughing. "I don't even like American men."

When there was a lull in the teasing, Nicola would turn on his reel-to-reel tape recorder and begin taping messages and snippets of funny interactions.

On the day before our trip each of us went through the weekly bath ritual that required heating the water, filling up the big aluminum basin part way, and adding some cold water to get to the right temperature. We were almost completely packed by late afternoon. My mother, my sister, and I had gone to the beauty parlor and my brothers to the barber.

The only thing missing was my dress. The seamstress had not yet delivered it and we were very worried. She was expecting a baby, and I was concerned that she had gone into labor and didn't have time to finish making my dress. I was so afraid I would not have anything special to wear on the big day.

Finally late in the evening she arrived, big belly and all, and delivered my beautiful raspberry crepe satin dress. I was ecstatic! It had turned out exactly the way I had designed it: a boat neck in the front, a low waistline, double pleats falling to just a few inches above the knees, and a low, V-shaped neckline in the back. I couldn't wait to wear my new dress.

The next morning I woke up before anyone else. My mother had left the door ajar to let in some of the cool night air. I could see the bright sun casting the shape of the opening on the wall across from my bed. So many Neapolitan songs and poems refer to the city as the most beautiful and romantic in the world: its sun as the brightest and its people as the most passionate. *Is this true? Will the sun shine as often and be as warm in New York as it is here?* My thoughts seemed frozen in time as I continued to look at the bright shape on the wall.

A few minutes later I heard my mother lift herself from the bed.

"Okay, everyone, it's time to get up!"

As soon as my mother spoke, we all bolted into action. That morning, our family dynamic was so out of the ordinary. No resistance to my mother's orders. No arguing amongst ourselves. No whining. No procrastinating.

"As soon as you are finished washing up, give me your toiletries and your nightclothes so I can lock the last suitcase."

We were ready in no time; except for Nicola who took his sweet time making sure his soap dish was properly sealed and his toothbrush in its plastic case. My mother probably wished we would be this cooperative and well-behaved all the time. But maybe there was hope for us. Now that we were going to America, we were going to be so much happier that perhaps we would be better behaved.

"By the end of today we will be on the other side of the world, in New York, with the rest of the family!" my mother said happily as she continued to get herself ready.

When I came out of our tiny bathroom, I glanced at the empty kitchen. It seemed so lonely without any people or furniture in it, but it was still filled with sunshine brought in by the four small windows surrounding it. *I wonder if our kitchen in America will be this bright and sunny?* I thought about all the times we would gather and laugh at the possibility of the kitchen tumbling away from the main building and rolling into the cemetery. I was excited about going to America, but I was sad about leaving behind everything familiar.

Poor Nicola had zero luck when it came to his feet. When he put on the pair of brand-new moccasins he was to wear on the trip, he discovered they were too small.

"I just bought those two weeks ago. How can they be too small?" asked my mother.

"I'm a growing teenager. Two weeks was a long time ago."

"Well, it's too late now, and you don't have a second pair of shoes. You will just have to stuff your feet in them and try to survive."

As soon as my sister was ready, she stepped outside onto the long balcony to keep an eye out for the airport car that was scheduled to pick us up. She was smartly dressed in a blue silk straight dress that she had made: tapered at the waist, clasped just behind her neck with a pear-shaped opening, sling-back heels, and a purse to match. She looked very elegant. She suddenly stepped back in the room and said, "The car is here. It's time to go."

Soon the driver came up for our suitcases. For the last time, we walked out of the large room that had been our home for many years. Dressed in our very best, we slowly filed down the outdoor staircase; down nineteen steps to the landing, a right turn and down eight more to the courtyard where the car was waiting.

The driver held the doors open as we climbed in. We felt so special. We had never experienced chauffeur service before. In fact, a car that size had never even been in our courtyard. The neighbors waved and stared at us from their doorsteps as though we were famous movie stars. The driver backed up a few meters, made a U-turn, and then we slowly drove out through the archway and into the street. We made an immediate right and more neighbors waved goodbye.

We veered a little left and passed the closet-sized candy store where we would go occasionally during the summer to buy shaved ice. The owner was a tall, elderly woman always dressed in black, with a big head of white hair. The only jewelry she wore was a wedding band and a gold chain around her neck with a crucifix. It was customary then in Southern Italy for women to wear black for the rest of their lives after their husbands were deceased. I wondered how much longer she would be there in that store.

Immediately on the left, we passed the wine store where my sister and I had gone every Sunday during the summer months to buy a half-liter of red wine and a one-quart bottle of *gassosa*, a sparking soda type of drink that we would mix with the wine to make our favorite drink for our Sunday meal.

The car veered right toward the piazza and I saw a man dressed in dark clothing walking close to the car. I wondered who he was. *Does he have a family? Is life a struggle for him like it had been for us?* Further up we passed fairly close to two more people who were probably walking to church. *Are they going to pray for a better life, like we have prayed for years and years? Do they wonder who we are and where we are going?*

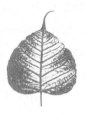

CHAPTER 65

FLYING TO NEW YORK

Once at the airport my heart started pounding. I couldn't believe that in a few minutes I would be inside an airplane. A machine that could fly way up into the sky, higher than birds, at a very high speed. There was so much excitement and newness in every step we took, there was hardly any room for conversation. Once on board we all checked our surroundings with meticulous care. Nine-year-old Pietro sat in the window seat, our mother next to him, and on the other side of the aisle Maria, Nicola, and me. Within the first few seconds, Pietro had every button, knob, lever, and everything else that could be moved or pushed figured out. My mother reprimanded him with her teeth clenched, trying not to be heard by the other passengers.

"Stop touching everything. You're going to make the plane crash," she said looking at all the buttons that Pietro had pushed. Soon an attendant came to explain to us the functions of everything. My mother relaxed. Pietro was not going to make the plane crash.

The flight from Naples to Rome, lasted not more than forty-five minutes or so, but they still served us a delicious breakfast. Foods we had never really had a chance to enjoy before: flaky croissants, butter and jams, fruit juices, coffee, and tea, with endless refills. It was Heaven.

In Rome it was raining really hard. Once the plane landed, each passenger was escorted into the airport terminal building by an agent holding an umbrella.

Before re-boarding for the next leg of the trip we were asked to wait on the tarmac for several minutes. The exhaust fumes became intolerable for nine-year-old mama's boy Pietro, so he started complaining profusely, as if there was something we could do about it.

Doesn't he know we're going to America? Does he expect the airline to funnel clean air directly to his highness' nose?

Soon after takeoff, they fed us another delicious meal with more things we had seldom had the chance to eat, including fresh tagliatelle. My mother worried that the tray of food was so overloaded we wouldn't be able to manage without spilling it on ourselves. Luckily, we all enjoyed our meals without incident.

In Lisbon, we deplaned for about forty-five minutes for refueling. My sister told me the ground hostess who checked our passports was tall and slender and wore an attractive uniform. With each passport she checked, she spoke the native language of the passenger. I was so taken by her self-confidence and sophistication, I decided right then and there that no matter what it took, one day I would be just like her.

During the last leg of the trip they fed us two more times. We were so used to eating just enough and only at regular mealtimes that it was very strange to see so much food being put in front of us. I hadn't gotten one crumb of food on my beautiful double-pleated dress, but it was wrinkled and that really bothered me. I wished I could iron it before landing. We were not used to looking less than impeccable in public. Of course, Nicola wished he could have slipped off his tight shoes at least once for relief, but he never did for fear he'd never be able to put them back on.

Returning from the lavatory, my sister sat in her seat again and said, "It's almost 11:00 p.m. in Italy. We should land in New York pretty soon." My heart leaped at the sound of that. It was still so sunny and bright outside. It was hard for me to imagine it was already dark in Italy and that our friends and neighbors were going through their first summer evening without us. I wondered if I would ever see them again as I pushed away some lingering feelings of melancholy.

My attention was quickly brought back to the present when the captain announced we would be landing soon in New York City! The adrenalin started pumping. Yes, soon we would start our new life. I wondered what was in store for us. At touchdown the passengers exploded in a round of applause, happy to be on the ground safe and sound.

As the plane taxied to the terminal we all sat quietly with our thoughts, trying to imagine what all this newness was going to be like: living in an apartment with several rooms, a television, a telephone, a washing machine, a refrigerator, a real shower, and hot water from a faucet!

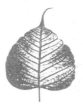

CHAPTER 66

BENVENUTI IN AMERICA

When we went through the passport check, the agent said the same words to each one of us.

"Something, something, something …"

None of us spoke a word of English, except for the usual obvious words that everybody knew, such as "yes," "mister," "OK," and "thank you."

Nicola, the professorial type, was the only one to give the agent a reply.

"I don't speak English."

When the agent got to me and said those words, I repeated them in my mind over and over to make sure I didn't forget them. I got goose bumps when I repeated them back to someone and learned the meaning of those words: "Welcome to the United States."

Our relatives had come to the airport in full force. Five big cars full of people waited for us! Before we even made it through the exit gate, Biagio and my father broke away from the group and started running toward us. Biagio ran into my mother's arms. My father lifted Pietro up in the air and then hugged and kissed all of us. We hadn't seen my father in a year and a half. We hadn't seen Biagio in over four years. My mother hadn't seen her brothers Domenico and Fidele in over ten years.

And of course, she hadn't seen her oldest sister Giacinta (Jenny) in over forty-three years. When my grandfather had repatriated the Cosentino family back in 1921, Jenny had traveled to Italy with her fiancé, Jimmy, just to get married in the presence of their respective families, and then returned to America within the same year. Many of the relatives who greeted us we had never met. Hardly any words were spoken, but we all shared lots of hugs, kisses, and tears of joy under the hazy skies of New York City.

Once this first emotional round of hugs and kisses subsided, my father officially introduced us to the relatives we had never met. We then slowly made our way to the parking lot where we all gathered around Aunt Jenny's car. Her husband, our Uncle Jimmy, opened the trunk. He took out a bottle of *anisette* and distributed shot glasses with a drop of the liqueur to everyone. He raised his glass and shouted, "Welcome to America!" followed by, "*Benvenuti* in America!" Everyone else repeated after him, "Welcome to America!" followed by a new round of kisses and hugs.

The relatives had decided ahead of time who would ride in which car. I ended up in a car with my great aunt Rosina and great uncle Nicola who had immigrated to America while we were living in Naples. They used to live near our farm in Basilicata. When my little brother Pietro was born I spent over two weeks with them while my mother was recovering from the birth.

When my great aunt Rosina took me back home, she carried me in a wicker basket on her head just because I had asked her to. I was four years old then and now at the age of 13, I was in a big American car in her company again, in New York City. Great Aunt Rosina's daughter Minicuccia (Donna) was in the front seat with me. Her husband, Vincenzo (Vinny) Labricciosa, drove. Donna and Vinny's one-and-a-half-year-old daughter, Grace, rode in the back with her grandparents, Great Aunt Rosina and Nicola.

The ambient sounds were very different in New York. The roads sounded very wide. The car rode smoothly with an occasional bounce that reminded me of a small ship riding waves as it floated down the road. The drivers did not beep their horns nearly as often as they did in Naples. I had heard that cars in America were very big but I had no idea that they would actually be this huge. There was so much room between the front seat and the back seat that baby Grace used it as a playpen. It was hilarious riding with Aunt Rosina and Uncle Nic. They were just as funny and as feisty as I had remembered them from my early childhood growing up on the farm.

It was dark when we arrived at Beech Street in Yonkers where we would be living. A number of our relatives had settled on this cul-de-sac as they immigrated over the years. Some of them had been living in New York for the past four decades. Others had immigrated during the more recent years while we lived in Naples.

Most were from my mother's side of the family. They had purchased apartment houses that they shared with other family members who were not yet homeowners. We would be living right across the street from Aunt Jenny in an apartment house owned by the Di Gennaros, Biagio's future in-laws. They lived on the top floor. Our apartment was on the first floor.

Uncle Dominico, my mother's youngest brother, owned the apartment building just two doors down. There he lived with his immediate family on the first floor. His in-laws, Great-Aunt Rosina and her husband, occupied the second apartment. His wife's sister, Donna, with her husband Vinny and baby Grace, lived in the third apartment.

We all gathered around a long table in their basement for dinner that night. The difference in the way things felt and sounded in Yonkers compared to Naples continued to amaze me. There was no echo whatsoever from being in rooms with high ceilings and tile floors like in Italy. Uncle Dominico's house was made of wood instead of stone and the rooms were small and carpeted, which made me feel like I was in a cozy and pleasant doll house.

Hearing all my relatives around me speaking my native dialect reminded me of my childhood on the farm, only we had suddenly been transported to a different land. Now the old language was sprinkled with words I didn't recognize like, "soda." At one point, my father asked Pietro and me if we wanted a soda to drink. Initially we were quite confused because in Italian, the word soda meant lye. We didn't really think that he would offer us lye, but he quickly corrected himself and called it by its proper name in Italian, "*gassosa*."

It was crucial in those days for immigrants to learn the most commonly used English expressions as soon as they arrived in America and include them in their own spoken language as frequently as possible. It gave them a sense of inclusion. That is how the language of the Italian immigrants came about. Most Italian immigrants at that time did not speak standard Italian to begin with, just the dialect they used in their region. When they were not familiar with the accurate vocabulary in Italian, they simply "italianized" the English word. One example is the names for the appliances they were now able to have in their homes. "Washing machine" became "wash machine-a," "refrigerator" became "friggitera," and so on.

After a long evening of good eating, drinking, and an emotional reunion-celebration, we walked home eager to discover where we would be living. My father carried Pietro who was already asleep. He opened the door and we saw our new home for the first time. It was smaller than I expected, but nicely furnished with many new things to discover: a television, a telephone, a refrigerator, a washing machine, a bathroom with a separate shower. The item that charmed me the most was the washing machine. No more helping my mother do the laundry using a scrub board.

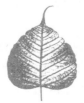

CHAPTER 67

FALLING IN LOVE WITH AMERICA

After a good night's rest we were up in a flash, eager to experience our first day in America. Our four-room apartment had about the same square footage as our place in Naples, but here the ceilings were low and walls separated the living areas. My sister and I shared one of the bedrooms and my parents the other. My three brothers slept on pull-out couches in the living room. Finally there was an adequate kitchen which also housed our washing machine.

Biagio and my father had already left for work and before we even started our exploration of the apartment, there came a knock on the back door. It was my future sister-in-law, Michelina, who lived on the third floor with her parents and her brother Bruno. With a cheery voice she said, "Good morning, everybody," and then repeated in Italian, "*Buon giorno a tutti.*" She had brought some Stella Doro breakfast cookies. She showed my mother how to use the stovetop percolator and together we sat down and had our first cup of American coffee.

"Here in America, most people drink their coffee in bigger cups than we are used to in Italy. It's less strong and they put a dash of milk in it. We Italian immigrants refer to it as 'brown coffee,'" she said. "When we make Italian coffee with the Neapolitan drip or the stovetop espresso pot, we call it black coffee or *demi-tasse.*"

"I don't care what they call it; it makes the house smell good and it makes me feel like an American already," I replied.

In Italy, only on very rare occasions did we drink coffee. It was very expensive and saved for special occasions. Now, here we were, enjoying big cups of coffee for breakfast.

Michelina also brought with her a can of hairspray. Much to my delight I discovered she was a beautician and was equipped to touch-up all the ladies' hair as soon as we were ready. Starting then and there, she became one of my best buddies for years and years to come.

Michelina gave us American versions of our names. My father, Raffaele, had become Ralph; Biagio had become Benny. My mother, Rosa, was now Rose; Maria was Mary; Nicola was Nicholas, Nic, or Nicky; and Pietro became Peter, Pete, and sometimes even Petey. I was the only exception. There was no American translation for Carmela. I was jealous and disappointed because I wanted an American name as well.

"Don't feel bad, Carmela. My mother doesn't have an American name, either. Her name is Emma in both languages," she said.

"For once, you don't get to have your own way," said Nicola.

"Who asked you, Nicola/Nicholas?" I replied.

After we had oohed and aahed over everything, Michelina, now Mickie, took her time answering whatever questions we had. She helped us unpack and organize things in the apartment so that we would be as comfortable as possible. She also helped my mother use the washing machine for the first time. She then told us for the next week or so we would not be eating a single meal at home. Our relatives would take turns hosting our family for meals. I was stunned. *I won't have to wash a single dish for a week!*

Our first lunch was with Mickie, and her mother, Emma, in our backyard. It was unusual for us to eat outdoors. Our living space in Naples hadn't included an outdoor dining area. Much to my amazement lunch was served on paper plates and it consisted of a sandwich instead of a fully cooked meal. I was in seventh Heaven with this American tradition, because it lightened my "Cinderella" duties around the house for sure. *It looks like I will have a lot of extra time on my hands with no laundry to do with a scrub board and no lunch dishes to wash. I love America!*

Mickie's mother Emma had developed a particular fondness for my nine-year old brother Pietro, now Peter, who was really good at impersonations.

"How do you like America so far?" she asked him?

"I really liked the man at the airport who stamped our passports," Peter said. He stood up, pushed his chest out trying to appear as official as possible, and gently slammed his knuckles on the table top to imitate the stamping of a passport.

"Welcome to the United States of America," Peter intoned in the deepest voice he could muster.

"Oh, Petey, you speak English already," she said, laughing.

All of us around the table were so amused by his impersonation, that from then on Emma would ask him to repeat the performance every chance she had.

Before lunch was over, Aunt Jenny who lived across the street, dropped in for coffee and dessert. One of the treats she brought for us turned out to be the most freakish food I ever experienced. Aunt Jenny put a bowl of something in front of me.

"Try this. It's called Jell-O and in America we eat it all the time. They say it's good for your bones."

The substance in the bowl wiggled and trembled every which way when I tried to cut it with a spoon. Initially I was afraid of it because it felt like it was alive, but I decided to try it and not be impolite. My sister noticed my discomfort so she reached over and chopped it up with her spoon, hoping to make it easier for me to eat it. When I put this stuff called "Jell-O" in my mouth and chewed on it, it wiggled like cold, clammy worms as it slithered down my throat. I had to concentrate hard to avoid vomiting. *How in the world do they think this is good? Even if it's good for my bones, I'd rather not eat it.* Jell-O almost ruined my infatuation with America.

Luckily what followed was a delicious Duncan Hines lemon cake with walnuts, homemade cookies, and brown coffee. I fell in love with America all over again.

The welcoming dinner parties in our honor went on for weeks. Every single Saturday and Sunday we were invited somewhere for an all-day celebration. The meals always started with an American cocktail, the highball (which almost all of us pronounced "eyeball"), and baskets of potato chips and Cheez Doodles. In Italy at the time, potato chips were sold only in single-serving bags and they were very expensive, so when I saw a generous amount of them in front of me, with more where those came from, I was a very happy camper.

At these parties I noticed how informally people addressed each other in America. Even children called adults just by their first names. It took me a while before I could do that comfortably. For us, it was unheard of not to address someone by his or her surname preceded by a Mr., Mrs., or Miss.

After the cocktails, the meal took a turn toward the Italian tradition: an antipasto consisting of prosciutto-wrapped breadsticks, olives, celery, other cured meats, and cheeses. Then came the homemade soup: chicken broth with tiny meatballs, a few other vegetables, and escarole. Fresh pasta, made from scratch, followed. Next came the assorted meats, usually meatballs, sausage, or short ribs that had simmered in the tomato sauce for the pasta.

The meal could have ended there, but we were actually just getting started. Now it was time to honor the American tradition. A short break followed in order to get the barbecue going, and soon grilled sausages, baby lamb chops, hamburgers, hotdogs, and numerous side dishes were passed around. After a fresh salad, seasoned with olive oil and vinegar, we thought for the second time, that the meal surely must be nearly over. But it was then that someone would emerge from the house holding a big pot with freshly steamed corn on the cob. In Italy, people ate corn on the cob only as street food, but we were now learning to appreciate it as part of a meal.

These extraordinary meals, fit for kings, were always accompanied by beverages, including good old American Coca-Cola, homemade wine from homegrown Concord grapes, or Gallo red jug wine served in plastic cups. In Italy, we had never been able to splurge on fancy foods or enjoy such overabundance. We had learned back home that coffee always sealed the meal, and nothing was to follow it with the exception of after-dinner liqueurs. But here we were having so much fun, we quickly learned not to fuss over culinary *faux pas*.

Finally it was time to dance. Someone would pick up an accordion and the music would start. Now that a real musician was among us rather than just self-taught accordion players, Nicola, now Nicholas, was of course the entertainer of choice. His repertoire was endless and he could keep us dancing for hours without ever repeating himself.

The first interruption of the dancing came with the dessert spread. This always included fresh fruit, stacks and stacks of Aunt Jenny's marvelous *pizzelle*, piles and piles of assorted homemade cookies, and what became my absolute favorite, homemade New York–style cheesecake. Then someone passed around Styrofoam cups of brown or black coffee. A *tarantella* involving everyone, including children, would energize the party—that is, until someone inevitably would notice that the watermelon had been forgotten, and so they sliced it and served it.

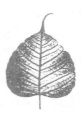

CHAPTER 68

A FULL SHOPPING CART

Lots of new American experiences swept me off my feet, and one of them happened to be our first trip to the supermarket, the A&P, on a Friday after dinner. In Italy, supermarkets were not common. Most people did their grocery shopping every day in small local food shops.

At the American supermarket, the first thing that shocked me was the sound of so many carts rolling in and out of the store. The second thing that amazed me was the size of the cart itself.

"This cart is big enough to hold you," my father said, laughing. "Do you want to ride while I push the cart?"

I declined.

It was a glorious experience walking up and down aisles packed to the brim with hundreds and hundreds of products to choose from. Benny and my mother pretty much stuck to the task at hand, consulting a shopping list and discussing meals for which certain ingredients might be needed. My father, on the other hand, took great pleasure in picking up item after item from the shelves for me to feel and identify.

At one point, he put a jumbo-size bag of M&Ms in my arms and asked me to guess its contents.

"If you can guess what it is, I'll buy you the whole bag," he said.

I recognized them immediately when I felt the candies through the plastic bag. "Picnics!" I shouted. That's what we called them in Italy, perhaps because the word picnic appeared on the package somewhere, so that's what we thought they were called. We had tried M&Ms once or twice in Italy, but we'd had to share one tiny bag among so many people that each of us was lucky to end up with one or two tiny candies.

My father laid the large bag of "picnics" in the cart along with other treats he thought we would enjoy. It was really wonderful to watch my father finally be able to splurge on his family.

"This is America," my father kept repeating as the cart got fuller and fuller.

At home once the groceries were put away, my father gave Peter and me a tour of the refrigerator, the cabinet where the snacks were kept, and the large bowl which was always filled with fruit, including bananas. With a big grin on his face, he said, "You can eat whatever you want, whenever you want, as long as you leave room in your stomach and an appetite for meals." My father had been waiting his whole life for the day when he could say this to us. My parents always made sure we never went hungry even when the money situation was dire. But, now they were finally able to indulge us with abundance.

Finally, we all joined the Di Gennaros in the backyard to enjoy the remainder of the pleasant summer evening. At one point I heard a jingling sound coming from the street. Both Mickie and her brother Bruno jumped to their feet and asked, "What kind of ice cream would you all like?" My father and Benny asked us the same question as if time were of the essence. What does that jingling sound have to do with ice cream? I wondered. And why was everybody in such a hurry?

As it turned out, both families were scrambling for the honor of paying for the ice cream. Bruno and Mickie rushed out of the backyard and won the race to the truck and soon returned with ice cream for everyone. Once we were all settled and enjoying our treat, Mickie told us all about the wonderful American tradition of ice cream trucks roaming through neighborhoods on warm summer evenings. *I love America!*

CHAPTER 69

DIRTY DISH WATER AND POST-CONVENT HAIR

The first few weeks we spent together in America as a family were blissful as we got to know each other once again. After all, the last time we were all together I was only nine years old. Lots of things had changed since then for each of us. Eventually though, our family dynamics reverted to familiar patterns. After a few family outings, Biagio, now Benny, who was quite a bit older than Maria and me, approached my mother with an opinion.

"I think you need to talk to Maria about the blue dress she keeps wearing."

"What about the blue dress?"

"I think that opening in the back makes her look cheap. She needs to fix it, because girls here don't dress like that," Benny said.

I couldn't believe my ears. *Girls here don't dress like that?* I was standing in the bedroom with the door to the kitchen open and overheard the entire conversation. *Oh my God! Who is he to tell Maria what to do?* Maria designed that blue dress from one of the latest fashion magazines, and he wants her to alter it?

I hadn't realized how wonderful the absence of a controlling male presence had been in my life. I had taken for granted the freedoms we had gotten used to in the last few years would continue even after my family was reunited. Suddenly I experienced that crushing, sad feeling of being controlled all over again—and in this case it wasn't even about me.

My sister and I had been ordered around by men, young and old, our entire lives, whether it was fair or not, just because we were girls and not boys. We had not been taught that women were on equal footing with men, quite the contrary. I felt outrage in my heart whenever we were faced with unfair treatment. *Was I born with this sense of justice in my blood? Why does it bother me so much? Whatever the case may be, I hope both my dad and this American "Benny" brother of mine haven't forgotten that I can scream, slam doors, and go on hunger strikes for days on end if they piss me off enough with their domineering attitudes.*

Although she was less rebellious than me, it still shocked me when Maria agreed to alter her beautiful blue silk dress. Benny was asking her to completely change this unique and elegant piece of art she had made with her own hands into something that would look plain and ordinary. What a shame.

At a later date, Maria finally did vent in the presence of the entire family over dinner. "People here don't understand anything about style or food. First of all, they drink coffee that looks and tastes like dirty dish water. Secondly, men wear their pants way too short. And worst of all, women are dressed and coiffed like they just stepped out of a convent a hundred years ago!"

No one responded to Maria's comments right then and there, but from that moment on, we all started referring to American coffee as dirty dish water and bouffant hairdos as the post-convent look.

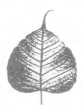

CHAPTER 70

PREPARING FOR SCHOOL

Between parties, gatherings, celebrations, and ice cream cones, the topic of school began to surface in our conversations. After all, fall was approaching and we couldn't go on partying forever. But this time I didn't have the melancholy feeling that I would experience in Italy before school started. I was looking forward to learning my most favorite language in the world and becoming a real American as soon as possible.

Based on the description of the rules and regulations, for the first time in my life I was actually looking forward to attending school. No school uniform, no licking your plate clean at every meal, no gender-segregated classes, no school on Saturdays. I could find nothing wrong with this. This was a sweet deal. I would even get to go home every weekend.

Soon friends and relatives began delivering bags and bags of clothes to our house. Although the few outfits we owned were stylish and of fine quality, we needed to have quantity to keep in step with the average American wardrobe. In America, people never wear the same outfit two days in a row, we were told. They don't necessarily clean the clothes between wearings, but the look must change every day. A lot of outfits I received were neither my style nor my size, but I was still grateful and excited by all the new wardrobe possibilities.

After lots of tricks and tweaks with the sewing machine by my talented sister, my suitcase was packed with five nice-looking outfits for the school week and I was ready to go to school the American way.

During the days leading up to our first week of school, everybody with whom we came into contact wished us good luck and reassured us we would learn to speak English quickly because we were smart. They warned us, though, not to get into arguments with Black kids because they were angry right now and were engaging in a lot of violence. At the time I knew nothing about the civil rights movement, so I couldn't understand the reasons behind the unrest, nor was anyone knowledgeable enough to explain it to me properly. The warning did not concern me because I couldn't speak the language anyway, so I failed to see how it would be possible to get into an argument with anybody. I had never met a person with black skin; therefore I was actually curious to see what they looked like. Considering how little I could see, their skin would have to be pretty dark and they would have to be pretty close to me in order for me to notice the contrast between the color of my skin and theirs.

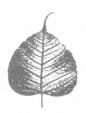

CHAPTER 71

LISTENING, LISTENING, AND MORE LISTENING

"Make sure the kids eat an American breakfast before you all leave. Ham, eggs, toast with butter, orange juice, bananas, American coffee, and whatever else they want. They need to go to school on a full stomach," I heard my father say to my mother before he left for the day.

My father and my brother Benny worked in construction, so as usual, even on our first day of school they had to leave the house at the crack of dawn. It was my Aunt Jenny's oldest daughter, my cousin Mary Marotto, who had volunteered to take my brothers and me to the residential School for the Blind. She was our closest relative who had a command of English and could drive.

It was cool and overcast that September morning in 1964. Mary, my aunt Jenny, and my mother sat in the front seat. The blind bunch sat in the back seat of the very spacious Cadillac. With our stomachs full to the brim, we teased each other about who was going to learn to speak English first. However, in spite of that we were full of anxiety. It felt as though we were moving to another new country all over again. So far we had spent time only with our relatives who spoke Italian, but on this day my brothers and I would face the real unknown.

We were shy and reserved when we met the school principal, the assistant principal, and the dorm staff. We had learned how to say, "Nice to meet you," but when the moment came and the school officials were shaking my hand, I forgot how to say it. I felt unprepared and stupid. However, they seemed so kind and unassuming that I soon felt reassured. Nicholas, the scholar, of course remembered the proper response. And Peter? He was too young to worry about such formalities.

After some discussion between the school staff and my cousin Mary, she conveyed to us that everything was set. There was no need for the family to worry. We said our goodbyes and of course, my mother couldn't leave without admonishing me not to misbehave and to do as I was told! *How can I misbehave and not do as I am told if I can't speak or understand what I am being told?*

The three of us were led off in different directions. The dorm staffer introduced me to Maggie, a girl a year or two older than me, who spoke Spanish. The assumption had been that Italian and Spanish were similar so I should have no trouble understanding her. Maggie seemed to have a bit more functional vision than I had at the time. She put her hand on my forearm and said, "*Vente.*"

I had always been good in math, so I put two and two together and decided that "*vente*" must mean "*venti*" in Italian (twenty). I was confused as to what the word "twenty" could possibly have to do with someone holding my forearm and encouraging me to go with her, but I followed. My math skills failed me, but soon a light went on in my head and I figured out that "*vente*" meant "*vieni*" in Italian, or "Come with me" in English. Yes, I will learn to speak English I thought, but apparently I must first learn to understand Spanish!

Maggie took me to the dormitory, showed me to the room I would be sharing with four other girls, and helped me unpack. My, oh my! Only five beds in each room instead of twenty-some! What comfort, I thought. Even more surprising, I soon realized this school was not just one continuous monastery-style building wrapped around a central court-yard. It was a real campus with many buildings for different purposes.

Next, we walked to the school building. In the entryway, Maggie showed me my locker where I would store my coat and books. Then she said, "*Ahora vamos en la biblioteca.*" Well, I thought, okay, "*biblioteca*" means "library" in Italian, so it must be the same in Spanish! Her hand is on my forearm, so the whole thing must mean "Let's go to the library."

As soon as she opened the door to the library, which was located right off the entryway, I experienced a feeling of delightful calm. The ceilings were low, the walls soundproof, and people whispered if they needed to talk to each other. We walked to a table in the study-hall room, and Maggie said, "*Sientate,*" while pulling out a chair and sitting down next to me.

I realized that I had already learned several words in Spanish — real progress for my English. She pulled a Braille book out of her bag and started reading. I had been at the school for less than an hour and I realized how totally unprepared I was for this experience. I wanted to know what was going to happen next but I had no way to ask.

A few minutes into my abyss of waiting, I heard the familiar sound of the class-hour bell. The room was well lit, and I was sitting close enough to the door to see how people moved about. Some of the students dashed out of the room with no trouble and I assumed they were those who had more residual vision. The rest slowly inched their way out of the room like blind snails. I had never seen blind people move around like that. *I wonder if they do orientation exercises here?*

Maggie stood up, put her hand on my shoulder and said, "*Espérame aquí. Ahora, tengo clase. Soy aquí en 50 minutos.*" And with that, she vanished. Each word she spoke was close enough to Italian that I was able to understand exactly what she meant: "Wait for me here. I have a class now. I will be back in fifty minutes."

I had no watch at the time, but I was sure the bell would indicate when the next class was over. Now I was really alone for the first time in America. Suddenly all of my worries surfaced. *What if I have to go to the bathroom urgently? Or what if I feel faint or nauseated? How do I ask for help?* My stomach tightened in apprehension. I tried not to think about it. I just wished I could have been better prepared. While I was lost in my thoughts, students who now had a study hall hour started pouring into the room, some holding Braille books, feeling their way around the room for empty chairs. The staff person at the desk would re-direct with a soft voice those who seemed hopelessly lost.

As soon as the next bell rang, everybody stormed out quickly, with plenty of bumping and "Excuse me's," along the way, trying not to run over one another. Again, bunches of blind people crowded the exit like a herd of sheep. I was shocked. I didn't know what to make of this. *It doesn't look like people have to follow many rules here compared to my school in Italy.*

Once the room was empty, the teacher on duty came over to me and in a cordial voice, said a string of, "blah blah blahs" ending with a question-mark intonation. What a treat, I thought. I was used to receiving orders and giving immediate answers to questions posed by school staff; but in this case, I didn't understand the question, nor was I equipped to give any answer. Total silence, a big smile, and a bewildered expression were all I could offer. *They can't punish me for not knowing English, can they?*

As I was about to despair, Maggie rushed into the room out of breath. She exchanged a few words with the staff member, then turned to me and said, "*Vamos a comer el lonche,*" or "Let's go have lunch." There came a slight chuckle from the staff member, but no indication that I understood what she had said. So Maggie tried again, "*Vamos a mangia mangia,*" (Let's go eat). Well, I certainly got the gist of that, but an uneasy feeling came over me. I was so confused and insecure about everything that I wondered if that chuckle had been at my expense. Nevertheless, I stood up, took Maggie's elbow, and followed her out of the study hall into the hallway, and out the door into the lobby, where we retrieved our coats.

We left the school building and followed the long pathway to the dining hall. As we were walking Maggie made a clicking sound with her shoes from metal caps on her heels, to keep them from wearing out. What was she doing wearing such shoes, I thought. They are so unbecoming! Metal caps on shoes in my mind indicated modest means or poverty. This sign of poverty surprised me. I didn't think there were any poor people in America.

I liked the layout of the school. I had always enjoyed being outdoors so much that having to walk outside from building to building was a treat. *I wish our school in Italy had had the same setup.* Moreover, I got to slip my newly acquired coat on and off several times a day, which was definitely a welcome distraction for a young teenager whose whole existence revolved around boys, new clothes, and hairdos.

I was finally free of school uniforms, which had kept my identity under wraps. Now I could experiment with different aspects of my personality by changing outfits and hairdos from day to day. I realized that in this setting, I actually had a blank slate. Nobody knew me so I could pretend to be whomever I wanted to be.

In the dining hall, Maggie showed me to my designated seat at a table for eight. On my right at the head of the table and standing behind the chair, was my brother Nicholas. It seemed ages since I had seen him last, although it had only been three hours. A few other boys had seated themselves at other tables with girls. What?? I screamed in my head. In this school, they were not a bit concerned about mixing estrogen with testosterone. The boys and girls were always together. *How fun and grown-up!*

Before I even had a chance to exchange a word with Nicholas, not knowing whether it was allowed, we heard a loud "ding," and everyone fell silent. Oh, this must be the time to say our prayers before the meal, I thought. A few seconds later, another loud "ding," and everyone sat down. Fantastic, I thought. Here, each person gets to pray or not pray, on his or her own terms. And that's the way it should be.

The dining hall was cozy and well lit, with wood flooring, big windows, and a low ceiling. I didn't smell any of the foods I was familiar with. The only eating utensils were a flimsy fork and a teaspoon for each person. No knife, no cloth napkin, and no water. There was, however, a full glass of milk at every setting. My God, I thought, it's true what they used to say in Italy: Americans drink milk with their meals even when they're grownups.

Unlike the school dining hall in Italy, students were very noisy here. Lots of talking, even with mouths full, and unladylike outbursts of loud laughter. Another Spanish-speaking girl named Dolores sat across from me, and she was already trying to converse with Nicholas. In the meantime, they placed a plate of food in front of us.

"It smells like the boiled cabbage mom used to feed the pigs on the farm," Nicholas said in Neapolitan dialect. I laughed.

Dolores kept repeating *"Como? Como?"* (What are you saying? what are you saying?)

"Lake Como is in Northern Italy. We're in New York here, don't you know that?" Nicholas answered, all in Neapolitan dialect.

I was the only one who could enjoy Nic's sense of humor. We could barely communicate either in Spanish or in English, so there was no way for us to share this humorous exchange.

I took one bite of each unidentifiable and tasteless item on my plate and left the rest. This was great; it felt good to be able to indulge in the luxury of not eating at last! I kept trying to find similarities with the school in Italy, but so far there were none. Once they removed the plates containing what Nicholas and I had thought was the first course of the meal, a lady came around offering something that ended with the sound, "cots." Some people were responding with "yes, please," while others with "no, thank you."

Nic immediately said, "That woman is saying a bad word."

I knew immediately where Nic was going with this. Nic's sense of humor was omnipresent. In the Neapolitan dialect, the word "cots" (*caz*) meant "dick." Being a typical teenager with hormones roaring through his body, his mind was never very far from his penis, I am sure. I started laughing uncontrollably, and now Maggie and Dolores were both trying to understand what was so funny.

At this point, I could barely say, "yes, please" to the lady with the "cots," so there was no chance that I could explain to Maggie and Dolores why Nicholas and I were laughing so hard. In the end the "cots" turned out to be apricots. We had never eaten canned fruit before, and for us it was a real treat to eat something deliciously sweet after consuming boring fresh seasonal fruits with every single meal for years on end.

"Mmm, this is a good palate cleanser," said Nicholas. "I wonder what they are going to serve next?" As soon as everybody was finished, the woman who had been introduced to me as the housemother came to the table and said something like, "blah, blah, excuse." At the sound of that everyone immediately stood up and started leaving the room.

"Maybe we're going to eat the rest of the meal in a different room," said Nicholas. Much to his surprise the male student assigned to escort him was soon at his side, as was Maggie at mine, so the meal was over. The boys and the girls left through their respective entrances, but they were soon together again outside for the recreation hour.

It was during this free time that one could see who was going steady and who was not. Nic and I were pleasantly surprised at how co-ed the school was. Maggie had a boyfriend who also wore metal-capped heels on his shoes. I felt sorry for him for sounding so poor and uncool when he walked. Many of the students gathered around Nic and me and tried to communicate with us. With help from those who spoke Spanish and my brother's humorous Neapolitan way of interpreting things, we made it through the hour with quite a few laughs.

We started the afternoon in the library, adjacent to the study hall. There we met with Mr. Cassaro, who was going to be our English teacher from 1:30 to 3:30 p.m., Monday through Wednesday. He spoke Italian, knew Braille, and was eighty-five years old. I didn't want to hold his age against him but I just couldn't imagine having a teacher who was older than my grandparents (who were almost all already dead).

We spent the first hour learning how to introduce ourselves and how to ask for a cup of coffee. The second hour, we read from a book written in Grade 1 Braille (each English word spelled out—not abbreviated by symbols). It was during this hour that I received the first two major blows to my confidence.

First, Mr. Cassaro explained to us that English is not a phonetic language like Italian, so the words are not necessarily pronounced like they are written. *Oh no, what does this mean?* Suddenly I realized that learning English was going to be much more difficult than I thought. But then he made matters even worse when he explained that standard American Braille books are written in Grade 2 Braille.

"What is Grade 2 Braille?" I asked.

"Grade 2 Braille means that words, or portions of words, are abbreviated into symbols rather than being spelled out," he said. He took my left hand and showed me the word "mother," spelled out, and then dot number 5 with the letter "M" next to it, which was the Grade 2 Braille abbreviation for the word "mother." A long pause followed. Nicholas and I were bewildered.

"Yes, it's going to be a long and tedious process," Mr. Cassaro said. "But you are young and smart, and I'm sure you'll get through it."

If I understood correctly, this meant we would have to first learn the meaning of the word in English spelled out, and then learn the abbreviated symbol used to read or write it in Grade 2 Braille. When I was finally able to swallow all of that, I felt like throwing up the lunch I hadn't eaten. This was not going to be an easy task, I thought.

I was going to have to learn my favorite language in the world by going through a labyrinth of twists and turns: first I had to learn Spanish so I could communicate with people through Maggie, then learn a whole new Braille code, and I had to learn it all from this man who was older than my dead grandparents! My demeanor changed and the color must have left my face because Mr. Cassaro asked me if I needed a break to get a drink of water.

During the two-hour session in the library, a boy stopped near our table to listen to Nic and me speaking Italian for a while. When he turned to walk away, I noticed the back of his jacket had orange or yellow letters so huge and contrasting that I could see them.

A few minutes before 3:30, the assistant principal, Mr. Walker, came to see us. He said hello and already I was confused about when to say "hello" and when to say "hi," so I ended up saying nothing. He informed us through our teacher that we would be sitting in classes with the ninth-graders. That was music to my ears because it meant I would skip middle school altogether.

But for Nicholas, it was a disaster. This school did not have the equivalent of the music program he had been enrolled in for the past several years and he certainly did not belong in ninth grade. Nic had already completed the equivalent of twelfth-grade academics at the conservatory of music in Naples.

At 3:30, Nic was summoned to the music floor to meet with the music director, Miss Toady, and with Miss Fisher, his piano teacher. I, on the other hand, was whisked away to a pottery class. I hadn't worked with clay since kindergarten. I did not like it then and I totally hated it now. I was always too fidgety to "Zen out" and enjoy making pottery. I didn't want to get my hands dirty and get stuff under my nails.

It was quite anticlimactic at the end of a long day filled with so many new and unexpected experiences. Miss Mattson, the pottery teacher, was completely thrown off-balance with my presence in her classroom. I supposed she had never been around anybody who was blind and did not speak English because she tried to communicate with me through sign language. She would mouth the words, point at things, and gestured to me as though I could see. Well, I didn't have the means to tell her I was blind and not deaf, so motioning to me was useless. And speaking to me in English was just as useless.

Strangely, all the teachers I had met in this school so far were sighted—not one blind teacher among them. Where are the blind teachers? I asked myself. Somehow I made it through pottery class as a deaf and dumb student. And I managed to receive a "very good" at the end of the hour. After all, shaping a piece of clay into a desired form only took a pair of willing hands.

After I had just learned how much more difficult it was going to be to master the English language and the American Braille than I had originally thought, Miss Mattson's class really finished stripping my self-confidence to the core. What's the matter with this teacher? I expected more from someone who had worked with the blind and visually impaired for years.

From 4:45 to 6:00 p.m., those who were fifteen and older with a special pass from their parents could leave the campus. At 6:00, dinner was served. It turned out to be even less appetizing than lunch, but it gave me a chance to laugh at my brother's comments. We wondered how Peter was doing. He was in lower school so we didn't get to see him. After dinner, study hall followed until 8:30 p.m., and then back to the dorm for the night.

The male students were allowed to walk with us to the front door of the dormitory. So much freedom, so much time, and opportunity for flirting and courtship compared to the strict rules and regulations at the residential School for the Blind in Naples. Here, people seemed unfazed by the whole process.

The girls my age acted silly and immature. They wore their hair in pigtails and wore girlish clothes. But they had one big advantage over me: they spoke English and I didn't! Before going to our rooms we all gathered in the living room, the only area that was carpeted and cozy with a fireplace and a piano. How fancy, I thought. We had nothing like this in the school in Italy. This is the good life!

Before long, someone came around handing out Styrofoam cups full of milk. "No, thank you," I was happy to say when she came to me. The last time I had been offered milk before bedtime was when I spent a month in the hospital during the measles epidemic when I was six years old.

Soon after the milk, somebody came around with a big plastic container full of cookies. They smelled really good, especially since I hadn't eaten much all day. I was not used to accepting treats without standing on ceremony, so I was hoping she would encourage me to take some when she came to me. But that's not what happened. She quickly moved on to the next person as soon as I said no, so I was left hungry and disappointed.

The girl next to me made no secret of her ferocious appetite for cookies. She scarfed them up in a hurry and washed them down with her milk in one gulp, followed by a full, open-mouthed burp and a long, "excu-u-u-se me." I was mortified. I wanted to hide under the carpet. The last time I had witnessed a living creature gobble down food like that I was standing next to my mother watching her feed the pigs on the farm. I guess I am standing next to an English-speaking pig, I thought.

Once we were tucked in bed and the lights turned out, a couple of my roommates continued talking gibberish for a while and then everything fell quiet. I stared at the ceiling in the darkness. I thought about my friends in my school in Italy and wondered how they were doing. I thought about all the things I would tell them in the next Braille letter I would write to them. It would probably take a whole volume just to tell them about my first day of school.

Before I knew it, the 6:30 a.m., wake-up bell was ringing and the second day in the American school was about to start. Not having to wear a school uniform and actually being able to wear a different outfit than the previous day was the first wonderful thing I had to look forward to.

At ten after seven, in no particular order, we all headed to the dining hall. As soon as we reached the entryway, I could smell real cooked food. It's true, I thought: Americans do eat a real meal for breakfast. The first thing I found waiting for me was a glass of delicious fruit juice. That alone was a treat for Nicholas and me. At our previous school they would never have served anything this sweet on a daily basis.

In the middle of the table was a big plate with a tall stack of buttered toast. The housemother quickly came around to serve coffee. The dining room server put a big bowl of something in front of anyone who said, "Yes, please." Nicholas said, "Yes, please," to everything.

I, on the other hand, accepted only black coffee with sugar and toast with salted butter. What I had learned to refer to as "brown coffee" with my relatives, and "dirty dish water" with my sister, here was just "coffee." For us it was watered-down coffee but I felt like a grownup to drink it out of a cup and saucer, instead of the usual *caffé-latte* bowl. Nicholas described what he was eating as crunchy flakes with milk and sugar.

"It tastes good. You should try it."

"No way," I said. "It has milk in it; that's for children."

After the cereal, they came around with plates filled with scrambled eggs and sausage. While Nic was eating his eggs, he said, "This is the type of big meal you're served before you get executed. I hope that's not what's going to happen to us!"

He described the taste of each item to me and told me whether it was worth accepting the next time around — not that I was planning to participate in this type of eating anytime soon. To me, it seemed unladylike to stuff one's face and express verbal enjoyment toward food. *Don't the girls find it embarrassing to be such gluttons in front of the boys?*

By 8:30 a.m., we were in the school building all lined up to file into the assembly hall, the girls and the boys on their respective sides, and the teachers following each line of students. The assistant principal stood at the podium and once everyone was in the room, said, "Please something." Everyone stood up and Maggie put my right hand over my heart and everyone recited what I assumed was the pledge of allegiance. I moved my lips, desperately wanting to look like I was participating, but the only word I was able to recognize throughout the whole thing was "America." Some announcements followed and then we were excused for classes.

Nicholas and I spent the entire morning sitting in one classroom after another, just listening, listening, and more listening, hoping that sooner or later we would start to understand something. Except for the two hours with Mr. Cassaro where we could enjoy a two-way conversation, the rest of the time we spent listening. By the end of the week I felt like my head had been encapsulated in a long, dark tube of gibberish.

Sitting in the Westchester County minivan that drove us home on Friday afternoon, I noticed that my teeth were clenched and realized they probably had been like that all week. I also felt as if my clothes fit loosely on me. Then I realized I had hardly eaten anything since I had left home.

As soon as we walked through the main door of the three-family apartment house where we lived on Beech Street in Yonkers, I could smell the wonderful aroma of homemade meals being prepared by the three Italian families. The cozy, delicious sensation that enveloped me was quickly vanquished by the harsh reality that my freedom to eat or not to eat had just ended. At meal times I could no longer say, "yes, please," or "no, thank you," to food. I had to eat and finish what was on my plate, which to me was torture no matter how good the food was.

"My American kids are home!" my mother exclaimed, smiling and meeting us at the top of the stairs.

"Do you still speak Italian or did you forget it already?" she asked as she hugged and kissed each one of us.

"What happened to you?" she asked me. "You look pale. Were you sick? Did they not feed you at school?"

"No, no, no," I replied, dismissing her concerns. "English is a difficult language to learn. I had to concentrate very hard; that burns a lot of energy."

After the initial greeting, Nic sat at the piano and announced our arrival to the neighborhood, while Peter and I went from house to house to greet people and proudly show off our new-found American selves along with the new words and expressions we had learned during the first week at school.

Riding back to school the following Monday morning, I wasn't nearly as excited and anxious as the previous week. I pretty much knew what to expect: gibberish, gibberish, and more gibberish. The only exception would be the daily two-hour interval with boring Mr. Cassaro, who made Nic and me read children's books because it was the only material he could find written in Grade 1 Braille. All other books were written in Grade 2 Braille. Peter, Nic, and I would eventually learn that code, but only after we had learned some English. I began to feel gloomy following this routine, day in and day out, without much progress to speak of.

One day after lunch, in my dismal state I heard the voice of a young Italian woman calling my name as she came toward me. She introduced herself as Miss Pane, Peter's English teacher. After a very pleasant chat, she walked away and I was left feeling even gloomier than before. Why can't we have a teacher like that, I wondered? We would learn English so much faster and it would be so much more fun. Everyone thought Peter was learning English faster than we were because of his young age, but in fact it was because of his teacher's young age and the methodology she was using.

Nic and I waited for Mr. Cassaro at the same table in the library every afternoon. Often a male student would stop near our table and just listen to Nic and me speak Italian. Then he would walk away. *I'm sure he has residual vision, because he walks around without hesitation in his step.* On one particularly gloomy day for me, he decided to stop and talk to us.

"Hello," he said. I was too low-spirited to react, so I let Nic do all the talking.

"Hello," Nic responded.

The young man took one of my hands and one of Nic's and said, "I'm Larry." I could see his hands were very dark and I assumed he must be one of the African Americans that I had been warned about. Unlike what my relatives had said about the current mood of African Americans, this boy did not seem angry. In fact, he was very nice. My small white hand looked very elegant cradled and wrapped in Larry's dark brown fingers.

"You are Larry?" asked Nic?

"Yes, and you?"

"I'm *Cumbá*" Nic responded.

"Give him your real name. He doesn't speak Italian. Why are you joking around with him like that?" I told Nic in Italian.

Larry seemed confused by my reprimand to my brother.

"You are Nicholas, right?" Larry said.

"Okay, I'm Nicholas and you are *Cumbà*," Nic retorted in English.

Larry burst out laughing, and with my residual vision I was able to see the contrast between his black skin and the most beautiful row of white teeth. I had finally met an African American person and he seemed very nice. I wished I knew what my relatives meant when they said the African Americans were really angry just then and there was a lot of unrest going on.

It would be a few years before I would really learn about the civil rights movement, slavery, and racial discrimination. In Italy, I had never heard disparaging remarks made about black people. We were only familiar with discrimination against the poor. Larry became one of our best friends and to this day he and Nic still address each other as "*Cumbà*."

When Larry turned to walk away from our table, I noticed again that he was wearing a jacket with something written on the back in big letters. What in the world was that? I wondered. Pretty soon, I started seeing some other boys wearing similar jackets. Then one day during the assembly hour a group of girls appeared wearing uniforms with very short skirts. They got on stage and started shouting words in a rhythmic tone, jumping around, doing some type of routine. It looked like a lot of fun and I wished I could be a part of it.

Sometime later I learned that the boys wearing those jackets were part of the wrestling team and the girls who jumped around were cheerleaders. Their job was to get the wrestling team hyped up the morning of each meet.

CHAPTER 72

PETER'S BIRTHDAY, AMERICAN-STYLE

During the second weekend home, we got to enjoy the first birthday party ever in our family. It had not been customary for us to celebrate birthdays in Italy. We had heard about the extravaganza around American birthday parties, so we waited with great anticipation for Peter's tenth birthday on the 27th of September.

"Is it true that all our friends and relatives are going to come here on my birthday and each bring me a gift?" Peter would ask.

"If you don't behave, nobody will come because I won't tell them it's your birthday," my mother would threaten.

But they came all right — and in full force! Each relative brought a box beautifully wrapped with fancy paper with a bow on top and a birthday card.

Our house was full of people and the gifts were stacked high. My brother Benny's future in-laws gave Peter his first snare drum, which was the beginning of his first drum set. I was mesmerized by the generosity and by all the festivities surrounding just one person. After this big to-do, I just couldn't wait for my birthday to come around.

Peter's phenomenal birthday cake and the assortment of Italian pastries had come from Caffé Puglia, the best Italian bakery in all of Westchester County. Thanks to this wonderful bakery many Italian immigrants, including my family, could finally afford to enjoy traditional Southern Italian pastries. For most of us back in Italy, the best we could do was to drool over these delicacies when passing pastry shop windows.

CHAPTER 73

PIANO LESSONS REVISITED

O ne midmorning toward the middle of the following school week, I was summoned to the third floor to meet with the music director. *What is this all about? Are they going to make me play the piano again? And who told them that I used to play the piano? I have been bombarded with enough disappointments. I can't handle even one more.*

As soon as I met Miss Toady, the director, she escorted me into a music room with two pianos. Miss Toady, who knew a few words of Italian from her extensive background in music, asked me to play something. My blood went cold. *What can I play? I don't remember anything. I thought I had left this nightmare behind.* I hadn't touched a piano since grade school, at least not to play classical music; and in a formal school setting with my upbringing, you just didn't play anything else!

Miss Toady repeated, *"Suona! Suona!"* (play!). After a few awkward moments, I shyly and gingerly played a few verses of the classic Neapolitan song "Santa Lucia." Since we had arrived in America, I noticed that everyone seemed to be familiar with this song, which is why I chose it to play for Miss Toady. When I finished she clapped and said, *"Brava, brava!"*

I was beyond confused. How could she find my silly performance commendable? After exchanging a few words of gibberish with Mr. Clark, she left the room. From what I could gather, Mr. Clark was now going to be my designated piano teacher. My heart sank. I had no desire to start this piano thing all over again. But without the ability to speak English, I was powerless.

Mr. Clark placed a sheet of Braille music on the ledger and sat next to me at the piano. He put my left hand on the first line of the music, and of course I knew he wanted me to play the right hand portion of the piece, then switch the process and finally play the two hands together like I had done for years. But as soon as I tried to read the first bar of the piece, I ran into some symbols that didn't make sense to me. *How do I ask him what this means?* Frustrated, confused, and embarrassed, I had no idea how to proceed. I'm sure he thought Braille was universal, just like print music. And I had thought the same until that moment.

Mr. Clark kept referring to the notes as A B C D E F G, rather than DO RE MI FA SOL LA SI (TI in English speaking countries) DO. I was totally lost. *Why is this happening to me?* After a few moments of nothing, he finally took my right hand, placed it on the keys and one finger at a time, he guided me through the notes I needed to play. His hands were soft and smooth. For sure, I thought, this man has never lifted a brick or used a hammer and a nail in his life. He smelled fresh and clean as if he had just showered and brushed his teeth.

His voice was pleasant and calm. *He seems calm, but can he lose his temper at any moment? Will he stomp away while yelling at me in gibberish and slam me into a corner for not following his orders? What kind of punishments do they issue here?* I was used to receiving harsh punishments but not without understanding the terms. Mr. Clark didn't lose his temper and with the help of a very kind American god, the bell rang and the lesson was over.

After the second lesson with Mr. Clark, it became clear that we were hopeless with each other, so I was handed over to Miss Fisher, the same teacher who had been assigned to Nicholas. Miss Fisher was young, energetic, and bubbly, and she spoke Spanish. But, was she aware I didn't have the same musical preparation as my brother? Did she have the same expectations of me? I could not read a whole page of Braille music to myself, memorize it, and then play both hands like Nicholas did. I had to first practice each hand individually several times before I could play them together.

Anyway, Miss Fisher was a much better match for me. She made sure that I understood everything she said and seemed to be in tune with my needs and personality. She also chose lovely piano pieces for me to learn. Suddenly I was enjoying playing the piano again, just like I did when I started taking lessons in second grade. After I learned the first piece she gave me, I was so happy; I wished I could play it for my grade school teacher just to prove that I could play well when I had the right instruction.

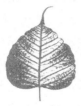

CHAPTER 74

GIRL SCOUT DROP-OUT

Within a week or so, another disappointment came my way. I found myself belonging to an organization that made no sense to me whatsoever. The first thing I disliked about it was the fact that once a week we had to wear a uniform. Every Wednesday this group of girls and I were expected to wear a navy blue skirt, a white blouse, and a wide sash with writing on it that looped diagonally around from the left shoulder down to the right side of the waist, and around the back. Occasionally we would go on stage during the assembly hour, recite some kind of a pledge followed by some more talking by some of the members. I had no idea what any of this meant. I couldn't have cared less and was bored with the whole thing.

One day instead of going to the dining room for lunch, we went to an outdoor area where our housemother, who was the leader of this organization, cooked hamburgers on the BBQ and served them with beans that were way too sweet for me. For dessert she put these round, fluffy, white things on a stick and roasted them until they were gooey, then put them on a piece of chocolate between two sweet crackers. Everybody was drooling and overjoyed with them.

I, on the other hand, really couldn't see what the big deal was. The chocolate was of poor quality and the roasted fluffy stuff tasted too sweet. None of it was worth the discomfort I was experiencing being out in the freezing cold with the imminent possibility of rain.

By the time my first year with this organization was over, my English skills were good enough for me to understand that I had been unknowingly enrolled in the Girl Scouts! Asked whether I wanted to rejoin, I immediately declined. I had spent enough of my life already wearing cheesy uniforms and being a good girl. I was eager to move on.

Chapter 75

Living in a Sugar Stupor

Pretty soon it was Halloween which was a totally new concept for us; celebrating the souls of the dead by dressing in scary costumes and going from door to door asking for treats. Then came Thanksgiving! I felt like we were quickly integrating into the American culture by celebrating all of these traditional holidays at the school. The day before we went home for the Thanksgiving break, we got to enjoy our first Thanksgiving dinner only three months after we had arrived in the United States.

It would be years, though, before a turkey would make its way into my mother's kitchen as part of this traditional celebration. When it finally did, she served it as a side dish: plain, dry, and without the trimmings. And it would take even longer before my mother was able to phase out the Italian food on this day and properly prepare a traditional turkey dinner. However, she never left out the first course of homemade ravioli, and she never gave in to learning how to make pumpkin pie.

Christmas was only a hop, skip, and a jump from Thanksgiving, and for us, it was truly a glorious time. The rhythm of life picked up speed. Big Christmas trees and elaborate decorations went up. Colorful lights appeared everywhere, indoors and out, hanging from trees, windows, rooftops, and doorways. An explosion of lights! I had never seen anything like it or even imagined that it existed anywhere.

Everywhere you looked were endless reminders that it was Christmas. There were Christmas parties in the classrooms. Cookies, cakes, candies, eggnog, and fruit punch were served and gifts exchanged. After a few days of all of this, I felt like my head was spinning — I lived in a sugar stupor. In the midst of this party frenzy, it seemed like not much time was spent thinking about the birth of Christ, the theme that dominated this holiday in Italy. I liked this American version much better.

At five o'clock one morning, as was traditional at our residential School for the Blind, we went Christmas caroling to the homes of the principal, the assistant principal, and other staff members who lived on campus. They served us cookies and hot chocolate.

On the last day of school, the students put on an elaborate Christmas show and we all received a gift bag filled with lots of treats, including a nicely wrapped box of chocolate-covered cherries. I didn't open the box right away, but when I did they smelled divine. I thought that finally I had hit the jackpot in the chocolate department. Each candy was elegantly nestled in its individual cocoon with the cherry stem still intact and hanging out of its chocolate coating.

I picked one up gently and anticipated the glorious flavor I would experience within seconds. I had eaten chocolate-covered cherries only once before in my life and had liked them so much. I felt lucky the opportunity had come around again. I put the treat in my mouth and almost immediately I was overwhelmed with disappointment. I quickly spit it out in disgust. The inside was so overly sweet and syrupy that I couldn't even bear to swallow it.

In Italy, chocolate-covered cherries were filled with liqueur and the chocolate coating was of the finest quality. They were sinfully delicious. Never in a million years did I think in the land of variety, abundance, and all possibilities, my most favorite treat in the whole world — good chocolate — would be impossible to come by.

When we got home for the holiday break our Christmas tree was already up with a pile of gifts under it. This was a first for us. Peter and I were in seventh Heaven. We spent all of our free time examining and shaking each box over and over trying to guess what was in it and who it was for. When we were home alone we would choose a couple of boxes that we thought might be for us and very carefully peeled the scotch tape, then opened the wrapping paper just enough to be able to squish in the side of the box and slip in one of our fingers to feel the contents. Sometimes we were lucky enough to recognize the item, thanks to our sensitive fingers. In the eagerness to find out more, sometimes the wrapping paper would rip, so we would mend it as best we could and hide the gift under all of the others to cover our tracks.

Each evening after an early dinner we as a family took turns receiving visitors or visiting all the other relatives with whom we exchanged gifts and holiday treats. The pile under our tree got taller and taller. We had never experienced anything even similar to this before. We felt as if we were living in a wonderland. We couldn't wait for Christmas Eve. My mother wanted us to wait until Christmas morning before opening the gifts, but we all protested and convinced her that on Christmas morning we were going to need time to get ready for church, so she relented.

Christmas Eve was glorious. It began with a long dinner with Benny's future in-laws, the Di Gennaros. They had prepared a feast honoring the culinary traditions from three different regions of Italy: Basilicata where we were born, Campania, the Naples region where we had lived for several years, and Abruzzi, the Di Gennnaros' region.

When it was finally midnight we were allowed to open our gifts. We took turns sitting on the couch being photographed as we removed each bow and unwrapped each box, revealing gift after gift. Our first Christmas in America was superb, magical, intoxicating. We spent the rest of the vacation visiting, eating, and celebrating. Then, on New Year's Eve came my birthday and a whole new pile of gifts appeared in our living room.

Only a couple of days later, it was already time to go back to school. I asked my father about Epiphany Day.

"You mean the old lady with the broom coming down the chimney?" he asked.

"Yes. Don't they celebrate Epiphany Day here?"

"Here in America it's a man coming down the chimney. It's Santa Claus! Have you already forgotten about all the gifts he left for you?"

"Well if I have to choose between the old lady and an old man, I'd say the old man is way more generous," I said.

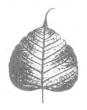

CHAPTER 76

CAN YOU SEE THE LIGHT?

Not too long after we returned to school from the Christmas break, everybody started talking about Valentine's Day. In America, it seemed to me there was no real pause between holidays. The girls were already going on and on about who they hoped would ask them to the Valentine's Day Dance, what they were going to wear, and what gifts they hoped to receive from their boyfriends. I found this confusing. In Italy, Valentine's Day was strictly reserved for unmarried couples who were romantically involved.

Another thing that confused me about Americans was their use of the word "love". I observed that the word "love" in the English language was a multi-purpose word used to express all sorts of emotions, not just to convey romantic feelings. I would hear people say, "I love your hair, I love your shoes, I love your bracelet." Even in romantic settings, I felt the word was overused. Every single time Maggie's boyfriend said goodbye to her, for example, he would add, "I love you." *What is the point in repeating it so often? He doesn't seem to really love her, because if he did he wouldn't get angry at her so easily and make her cry so often.* But I supposed this was part of the American culture and I was living and learning.

When the "Big Love Day" finally arrived, it was "Happy Valentine's Day" to anyone and everyone. It seemed like everyone was walking around with a fancy, heart-shaped box filled with chocolates of all different shapes and flavors. I had learned the hard way not to stand on ceremony as we did in Italy when someone offered me a treat, so I accepted readily if someone wanted to give me chocolate. But I was disappointed with every flavor and shape I tried. Nevertheless, I liked this abundance of chocolate. *If it were only Perugina Chocolate, I would be in seventh Heaven!*

The school day was cut short so all the students would have extra time to get ready for the Valentine's dance. Even dinner was served early so the kitchen staff could remove the tables and chairs, turning our dining hall into a ballroom. Colorful paper streamers emphasized the festiveness of the occasion. My favorite color, red, seemed to be everywhere.

In my dorm room, the girls were very chatty about the fancy dresses they were putting on. They eagerly walked around the room so we could all examine each other's' outfit. Most of the girls wore puffy, glittery party dresses, spiked heels, and bouffant hairdos. Everything was too cheesy and flamboyant for my taste, but they were having a good time, and that's what mattered. I felt very comfortable in my understated, but fashionable Italian outfit. I had learned by now that Americans "loved" compliments and if I didn't make a nice comment about each dress, it would mean I didn't approve.

"Very beautiful," I would say to each girl as she passed by my bed.

Splashed in cheap cologne and dressed in their best polyester suits, the boys walked over to the girls' dorm with corsages in hand to pick up their dates. As each one arrived, the housemother would ask, "And who are you picking up, sir?" The boy waited in the living room for his date to join him. He would pin the corsage to her dress and they would walk romantically together to the now-transformed dining room.

I walked to the dance along with the other dateless girls. For those with boyfriends or girlfriends the fairytale seemed complete. But the rest of us were left wondering what romantic luck waited for us in the stars.

I was noticing constant contradictions in this culture. American kids were allowed to act like grownups in many ways, but in some other ways they were controlled as if they were children. The school had a rule requiring that when dancing to slow songs there had to be enough distance between the two dancers so that light could be seen. Some of the older boys, to make fun of the rule, brought flashlights to wedge between themselves and their partners. This would oblige them to dance very close together to keep the flashlights from falling.

The Assistant Principal was the chaperone for the evening. Occasionally you could hear him shouting over the music, "Too close, Jim! I can't see any light!" *How tacky and embarrassing.* The right answer though, quickly put an end to the awkward moment.

"You must be blind like me, Mr. Walker. Can't you see this flashlight?" Jim shouted back.

The Assistant Principal took the joke well and the gala continued with many laughs. Halfway through the evening, when a slow tune came on, I could see a tall figure coming toward me. He definitely had quite a bit of residual vision, because he took my right hand without fumbling and asked, "May I have this dance?"

From his voice I recognized him as an older Black student who had said hello to me several times around school. He was so tall he had to fold himself in half to get to my face level. At the end of the song he held me tight for a moment and then walked me back to my chair, thanking me for the dance. He formally introduced himself as Jonathan. And before I knew it we were dancing together for almost every song. During the last dance he took off his tie clip, put it in my hand and said, "I want you to keep this to remember me by. It's all I am allowed to give you." At the end of the night Jonathan thanked me for a wonderful evening and walked away.

All of the other boys walked their dance partners or dates to the girls' dorm, but not Jonathan. I wondered why. It would take me years to learn that the school policy strongly disapproved of interracial dating.

CHAPTER 77

THE HONEYMOON'S OVER

Mr. Cassaro called in sick one day just a week before Easter break. Nic and I were not exactly disappointed. Our time with Mr. Cassaro had not been very productive. We were finally making some friends and our English was improving steadily — but certainly not because of the children's books written in Grade 1 Braille that Mr. Cassaro required us to read.

When we returned to school after Easter break, we were informed that Mr. Cassaro had died and there would be no replacement. However, we would still spend those same two hours in the library learning on our own. That is Nicholas reading and learning, and me on the other hand, playing with my hair and experimenting with makeup. I was certain if Nicholas ran across anything he deemed important for me to learn, he would tell me about it.

By now I had spent enough time in America to realize that learning here was considered very optional. If you learned a lot, you were rewarded with good grades, but if you didn't you weren't crucified for it. You wouldn't be held back for an entire grade for failing one or two subjects; you would simply repeat the class you hadn't passed.

Toward the end of the school year, Nicholas began acting very frustrated and started complaining to my mother that he wasn't learning or accomplishing anything. My mother, a very intelligent woman but only somewhat literate, never questioned Nicholas' words when it came to academic matters. Even though my mother loved being reunited with the extended family in America and having extra money in her pocket, her blind children's education came first above all. My brother's dissatisfaction with his schooling put her on notice.

On the last Sunday before summer break, the school held its annual picnic. It was an opportunity for families to visit the school and interact with the staff, teachers, and other students. The festivities included music, food, an auction, and a raffle with an impressive selection of prizes. My entire family attended, including some of my aunts and uncles. We purchased so many raffle tickets we were not surprised when my mother and my younger brother Peter won the first and second prizes: a money tree with 100 one-dollar bills and a portable color TV. We were ecstatic because a color TV was a huge thing in the mid-60s, especially for a low-income family!

The party had been a happy occasion as far I could tell; however, the next day I overheard my mother talking to my father in the kitchen.

"Did you see those blind kids at the school, how ill-mannered and socially clumsy they were?"

"Why? What was wrong with them?" responded my father.

"Everything was wrong with them! It looks like nobody is teaching those kids anything. They don't sit up straight. They don't look at people when they are talking to them and most of them have terrible table manners. It seems to me like these kids are neglected both at home and at school. Why is that?"

"I don't know why it's like that, but I'm sure our kids will be fine."

Oh my God, I thought, I've never heard my mother complain about America before. *Is the honeymoon with America over?* Then, she continued.

"Something isn't right. We've been here almost a year and outside of the family, they have made no friends. In Italy, it seemed so easy for them to get to know kids their age when they came home from school. Here it's not the case. Sighted kids here don't want to associate with them."

"It's not that people don't want to associate with them, but here it's difficult for young people to get to know each other outside the school setting. There's no *piazza*, no *passeggiata*, and no cafés where it's easy for young people to meet each other."

"Well, I don't like it!" my mother said.

Since many of our relatives lived practically next door they often came to visit. I heard my mother bring up this topic again and again with my relatives. They tried to reassure her that things would work out eventually.

"We know that in Italy blind people get financial assistance once they turn 18, but we don't know about how it is here in America. Maybe they will get assistance here as well if they need it," said one of my uncles.

My mother listened but she was not convinced. Each day she seemed to become more and more resolute and more convinced that her blind kids would not get a good education in America.

"I don't think this is the right place for them. I'm taking my kids back to Italy where they're going to grow up better educated and more socialized. At least in Italy at the age of 18 they will have a guaranteed stipend to keep them out of poverty. They will receive assistance whether they need it or not." She raised her voice as she said, "Here, they are going to end up as blind beggars and they're going to look the part too!"

"Maybe one way to do it would be to send the kids back to Italy for the school year but bring them back to America for the summer," one of the relatives would suggest.

"That's an option," my father would say.

"No, that's not an option. We've lived through that before. I'm never going to be far away from the kids again," my mother would respond.

"But they're older now. It would be different," somebody else would reply.

"No, no, no. The only way to do it is for me to go back with them. Rent an apartment near the school so they can come home every day if they want to."

Come home every day if we want to?

My heart leapt with joy when I heard those words. We would have an apartment near the school! How fun! That's one of the most expensive areas in all of Naples! I could see myself walking to and from school every day wearing nice outfits that would make my classmates jealous. After all, I would be a day student — an American student, for that matter. The school would never dream of imposing a uniform on me anymore! I would be able to enjoy a different status now.

But after my silly mind swirled around this glorious existence, it suddenly landed on a grim reality: academically, I would now be so far behind my former classmates there was no way I could still be in the same class with them. I was sure that by now they were already reading Dante's *Inferno*, while here I was still reading *Jack and Jill Went up the Hill*. Who was I kidding? School in Italy was serious business. It was impossible to learn anything half way and get by with it. Multiple choice and True/False tests were nonexistent. Did I really want to go back and study that hard again? I was conflicted.

One thing I knew for sure, though: I wanted to keep having fun and enjoy more freedom even if it meant growing up a little less educated. The only ones who were sure about going back to Italy were Nicholas and my mother. The topic dominated many family conversations throughout the entire summer of 1965, and finally it was decided that by the end of the school year in 1966, my mother and the three blind kids would return to Italy.

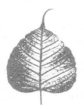

CHAPTER 78

DREAMING AT MY OWN PACE

Thanks to our much-improved communication skills, Peter, Nicholas, and I became more socially involved during the new school year. Nicholas with his sexy Italian accent, musical talent, and debonair personality became the new darling of the school. Girls followed him everywhere. Nicholas here, Nicholas there, Nicholas, Nicholas everywhere. Wherever he went, there were girls ready to charm him. And he charmed them.

Much to my total shock, I was asked to join the cheerleading squad for the wrestling team. "Who, me?" I asked.

"Yes, you," the squad captain replied.

"But I don't speak English well enough, and I don't know the cheers."

"You speak English well enough and we will teach you the cheers, don't worry," she replied as she handed me my uniform and the mysterious letterman jacket that I had seen people wear when I first came to the school. Now, I finally knew what it represented.

The girls on the team taught me the words for each cheer along with the physical routine. I was blissfully happy. Bouncing around on stage in a micro-mini uniform cheering on the wrestlers before each meet became my new passion. I was not willing to give it up for anything, not even going back to Italy to become better educated.

During the Christmas vacation my mother provided us with an update on her plan to return to Italy. I told her immediately that I didn't want to go back. Peter remained silent. I'm sure he was happy with his current easy-going school arrangement.

As for Nic, it was a little more complicated. The academic curriculum in Italy was extremely demanding. It would take a monumental amount of work for us to make up for lost time. He paced around the apartment with his hands clasped behind his back like an eminent philosopher in deep contemplation. He was trying to find a solution to the most mystifying problem of the ages. We talked about it amongst ourselves several times during the Christmas break. And all three of us, for different reasons, were developing cold feet about the prospect of returning to Italy.

My mother knew that Nicholas was the one who had lost the most by interrupting his music studies and coming to America, so she left it up to him to make the final decision. Before we returned to school in January, Nic told my mother the three of us had decided to continue our studies in America. And he told her he wasn't going to continue at the New York Institute for the Education of the Blind.

"What do you mean you aren't going to continue at NYIEB? What are you going to do instead?" asked our mother.

"I'm going to transfer to Lincoln High in Yonkers, because with my background, they will allow me to graduate from high school much sooner than at the Institute," Nic replied.

"Are you sure you will be able to do it? Who will read you the material? Do they have Braille books?"

"Don't worry about that. I'll figure it out."

My mother responded with a long sigh. "I hope you know what you are doing."

It was highly unusual in the 1960s, for blind students to be mainstreamed in public schools, but Nicholas was determined to do it. The school officials reviewed Nic's academic records and allowed him to complete high school in two more years rather than three.

He then went on to graduate from Michigan State University with a bachelor's degree in Romance Languages, and one year later earned a certificate in interpretation from Georgetown University. He was immediately hired as a professional interpreter with the Common

Market (now the European Union) in Brussels, Belgium, where he resides today. Music is still Nic's favorite activity and he often plays jazz keyboard with bands or as a solo performer.

Meanwhile, Peter and I continued our education at the New York Institute for the Education of the Blind. Peter was making speedy progress learning English and was beginning to make new friends. I, the least ambitious of the three, was happy to keep my grades just above average so I could coast through school undisturbed, while I assembled and disassembled my dreams at my own pace.

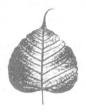

CHAPTER 79

A SOBERING MOMENT OF TRUTH

During the summer months of 1966, a little job came my way. A new friend of the family named Joe, also an Italian immigrant, owned a luncheonette in downtown Yonkers. He offered me a job washing dishes from 7:30 in the morning to 4:00 in the afternoon. I would be making $20 a week, plus an occasional tip. This was my very first job and I felt rich earning my little salary. I had to overcome one major hurdle, though. I didn't feel 100 percent confident walking to and from the luncheonette by myself.

I had walked downtown arm-in-arm with my mother on many occasions so I knew exactly where the luncheonette was located. But could I walk back and forth by myself? I decided right then and there that I would not admit my insecurities to anyone and risk losing my first job. "Can you walk from here to Main Street by yourself?" Joe asked me as we sat at our kitchen table with my mother.

"Of course I can. I know my way. I can get there," I said.

"She walks with me downtown all the time," my mother said to Joe. "She knows her way around. It will be good for her to have a little job for the summer so that she can start earning some money. It will keep her out of trouble."

Joe and my mother both chuckled.

Before I started my job at the luncheonette the following Monday, my mother and I walked back and forth to the place a few times to make sure I could really get there safely by myself. While my mother had given me the "go-ahead" in front of Joe, I still had to prove to her that I really could do the route safely.

Luckily it was overcast on both days when we practiced, so I didn't have to struggle with the glare from the sun which often created deceptive shadows. Practicing the route with my mother walking a few yards behind me instead of next to me unexpectedly made me feel less secure. Without my mother walking by my side my route to work suddenly seemed more complicated than I could have imagined. Of course I tried to keep all of that to myself, because I didn't want to risk losing the job.

To get to the luncheonette, I had to walk out the front of my apartment building, cross Beech Street, and walk through a small parking lot before I reached several flights of stairs leading to the street below. Stairs leading down were problematic. I couldn't see well enough to locate the first step unless the lighting provided a strong contrast, so I often had to rely on other visual clues such as the dark patch of grass growing to the right of the railing.

After navigating the multiple flights of stairs I made a left on Oak Street. At the first corner I crossed Oak to begin the four-block stretch on Park Hill Avenue that would take me to the luncheonette.

As for the route back home, the most difficult part was still the multiple staircases that now presented a different challenge. While light created shadows on each step that I could see, there were often a bunch of school kids sitting around on the first flight of stairs, creating a hellish obstacle course. Because I couldn't see exactly where to put my feet, one tiny mistake and I would become a laughingstock. That would be a nightmare for me.

Thankfully I did all our practice runs perfectly so my mother's mind was put at ease.

"You did everything right, but you still have to promise me that when it's time to cross the street you will wait if you are not 100 percent sure it is safe," my mother said.

"I promise."

The morning of my first work day I awakened feeling like a grownup. I, too, now could be out of the house all day, come home by early evening and be able to say to anyone who bothered me, "I worked all day. I'm tired. Leave me alone." I quickly thought about the next Saturday when I would receive my paycheck of $20.

I suddenly remembered a promise that I had made myself ten years prior when I tasted chocolate for the first time. I had experienced such an uncontrollable urge to have more that I decided right then and there, that I would spend my first paycheck on chocolate, and chocolate alone. But now I was a teenager and there seemed to be so many other things I was salivating over: clothes, shoes, purses, stylish sunglasses, and makeup. Spending $20, even on good chocolate, seemed like such a waste.

I was very nervous when I walked out of my apartment building that Monday morning. Luck was not on my side as it was a bright, sunny day. I had to do the route all by myself with the sun casting lots of unpredictable shadows confusing the way I could see things. I prayed profusely on the way down to the luncheonette hoping not to make any mistakes. Each decision point on my walk felt like playing a game of Russian roulette.

I made it down the multiple flights of stairs successfully, but once at the corner of Oak Street I noticed that all the ambient sounds were louder than ever. I finally realized it was a work day, so of course it would be noisier than when we had practiced the weekend before. Today I was assailed with a lot of street racket and beeping car horns. *Am I doing something wrong? Are they beeping at me?*

I stood at the corner of Oak and Park Hill waiting for a quiet moment to cross the street, which was the only method I had learned. The longer I stood there, the more nervous I became. When a quiet moment occurred and I could see the crosswalk was clear, I started walking. Once I made it to the other side of the street successfully, I felt re-encouraged.

By using the sliver of functional vision I had, an enhanced sense of hearing, plus years of orientation exercises at the School for the Blind in Italy, I was able to move about in familiar surroundings with the confidence of a sighted person. But now I began experiencing the flip side of my ability to fool people. In this situation it certainly was not working in my favor.

I made it all the way to the corner of Park Hill and Main Street without further incident. I was ecstatic.

The more I walked back and forth to work, the more confident I became with doing the route. One day I left work at 4:00 p.m., glad that it was overcast as it often is in New York during the summer. I carried myself with the make-believe confidence of a top model: long strides with toes pointing outward. I was wearing a straight red skirt, black and white striped shirt, patent leather sandals, with belt and purse to match. And of course, every strand of hair in place with the most stylish pair of sunglasses on my face. I projected the image of someone who could see perfectly and had the world wrapped around her little finger.

As much as I hated to admit it, my mother was right. It was true that my brothers and I had not really made any friends outside the School for the Blind. In Italy, I had lots of friends outside of the school. In America, sighted kids our age seemed to be very cliquish and ill at ease around blind people. I thought to myself how nice it would be to have a friend to do things with and not have to go straight home after work.

As I approached the first street intersecting Park Hill Avenue, I could see the white lines of the crosswalk and I could hear cars idling on my left. I stepped off the curb to cross without any worry. Once on the opposite corner, I scanned my way forward in an effort to identify any obstacles. I saw what I thought was a man standing in the middle of the sidewalk. To me it looked like he was wearing dark pants and a light colored shirt. I saw something dark above his torso, which I assumed that it was his head. When I got closer to him, I had to decide whether to pass him on the right or the left. I heard him speaking to someone, but couldn't see where that person was standing. I decided to pass him on the left and hope for the best.

Suddenly I found my mouth slamming straight into his left arm, which was stretched out and resting on the wall of the building. In pure surprise, he stepped back and with a super-snotty attitude said, "What's the matter with you? Are you blind or something?"

I stared at him indignantly and said, "Yes, I am. Do you mind?" I proceeded to pass him, stepped to my right, and continued down the sidewalk. Within a step or two I slammed into a ladder that was leaning against the same wall. I was mortified. I nearly melted in my clothes from shame and embarrassment. Somehow I found the courage to walk around the ladder and continue down the street, trying to project an attitude that it was other people's fault for leaving things in my way.

Perhaps I should have realized from multiple clues that the little bit of functional vision I had was diminishing. As a teenager, I was extremely fussy about my hairstyles. I was always literally pressing my nose against the mirror, trying to see what effect my ever-changing hairstyle had on my face. I noticed occasionally that my face looked somewhat fuzzy, but I attributed that to the poor quality and the small size of the mirror I was using. Never did it cross my mind that my little bit of vision was gradually slipping away from me.

The words "degenerative disease" had never registered in any of our minds when my two brothers and I were diagnosed with Retinitis Pigmentosa as children. My parents were in such despair when they found out three of their five children were blind, the eye doctors chose not to dwell on how the degenerative part of the disease would manifest later in life. My parents preferred to rely on the false hope that one day we would be able to see.

"Doctors come up with new things all the time. I'm sure that one day our kids will be able to see," my father would say to my mother, hoping to relieve her of some of her grief. Once we immigrated to America he was even more sure of himself.

"We are in America now. This is where they find solutions for everything, and anything is possible."

Since my parents had not been willing to accept the whole truth about Retinitis Pigmentosa being a degenerative disease, we kids had been growing up unaware of the details of our eye conditions. The truth was that my blind brothers and I, ever so gradually, were losing the little bit of functional vision we were born with.

My brother Nicholas experienced quite a sobering incident himself. One day he was out having a drink and a cigarette with our good friend, Larry Bunn. Larry was our first African-American friend, whom we had met before we even spoke a word of English. That day, when Nic was finished smoking, he pressed his cigarette butt in what he thought was a dark ashtray on a white table. Instead, it turned out to be Larry's black hand.

Larry exploded in an extremely loud squeal as he experienced excruciating pain. Nic apologized profusely once he realized what he had done. Larry was blind himself so he knew only too well these things could happen. Luckily the incident didn't damage the friendship. Larry proudly wears the scar to this day and loves to tell the story.

Using a white cane and coming to terms with our blindness would have been the right thing for us to do all along. Instead it would be more than a decade, well into our post-college years, before we would begin living responsibly with our disability.

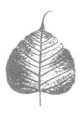

CHAPTER 80

MY FIRST ENCOUNTER WITH A PREDATOR

My job at the luncheonette was quickly coming to an end as the new school year was just around the corner. I was looking forward to spending just a little bit of the money I had made on new outfits to wear to school.

One or two days before my job at the luncheonette was supposed to end, Joe the owner, asked me to help him organize some shelves in the back of the restaurant. Right off the bat I thought it was odd that at the end of the day, minutes before I was supposed to leave, he would ask me to begin working on a new project. I followed his orders. Once we were in the storeroom, he closed the door behind him and locked it.

"Don't worry, this won't take long. Don't be afraid. Nobody comes back here anyway, but I have a gun in case they do. I can protect you," he said, smiling as he moved closer to me. As I heard his words, I nearly melted with fear and confusion.

I thought to myself, is he serious about having a gun? Why does he have a gun? He wrapped his arms around me, tried to kiss me, and pushed my right hand onto his belt buckle, urging me to undo it. How disgusting I thought, what is he doing? I was infuriated and repulsed! How dare he do this? I thought. He's almost my father's age!

I twisted my way out of his grip and nearly stumbled on a blanket he had put on the floor. I rushed to the door, unlocked it, and slammed it behind me. As I was hurrying away I ran into the counter with the left side of my body. I was in excruciating pain, but the rage and disgust from what had just happened kept me moving as fast as I could.

I grabbed my purse and ran out the front door. I was fuming. I wished I could get into a car and drive off, with tires squealing and screeching to express my frustration. But instead I was trapped in my blind body unable to channel my riled up emotions to my satisfaction. I had to pace myself. I had to scan each small section of my path forward before I put one foot in front of the other to make sure I didn't run into anything. My inability to move quickly was burning me up inside. *I hate being blind!*

The walk back home that afternoon was a nightmare. I knew for sure what had just happened made no sense to me whatsoever. If I were to mention it to my parents, it would make even less sense to them. After all, Joe was a friend of the family. It would sound unreal to them. I was disgusted and bewildered by his actions.

Why would a man nearly my father's age hug me, try to kiss me, and encourage me to undo his pants? I had no idea that men like that existed. I thought before two people arrived at the hug and the kiss part, they went through a lengthy courtship. But even if he had engaged in a long courtship, or any courtship at all, I wouldn't have responded to his advances. There was nothing about this man, or any man like him, especially in his age group, that I would ever find attractive. Why was this fact so obvious to everyone but him? And what about his wife? How could people love each other enough to get married but then not be true to each other? Don't married people love each other forever? Why did life suddenly seem so sad and ugly?

I felt completely uncomfortable sharing the truth with my parents. Instead, I told them that the job ended a couple of days early because the new dishwasher Joe had hired wanted to start right away. I was on pins and needles for the remaining days before we resumed the academic year at the residential School for the Blind. I was afraid Joe might stop by to visit with the family and torture me with his presence. Luckily, he never did.

It took me years to learn that people like him are called predators. I wish I had realized what his full plan was on the spot, because I would have gladly punched him in the teeth with my right fist and kicked him in the nuts with my right knee and taught him a lesson that would last a lifetime.

CHAPTER 81

AGAINST ALL ODDS

Our immediate family was shrinking a bit. Benny and Michelina had married in March of 1966. They had remodeled and settled into the apartment just above us on the second floor of the Di Gennaro's apartment house on Beech Street. The newlyweds were wedged between both sets of in-laws, creating the perfect setting for raising their children with free babysitting. Staying together as a family this way was common for immigrants as they shared resources and kept the money in the family. My brother and his bride were continuing the deeply rooted traditions from the Italian farm communities where the work of each member of the group was indispensable in ensuring the success of all.

We had been in America for almost three years now and like every immigrant family, we were doing all we could to realize the American dream. Every member of my family who was able to work had a job, and we were all contributing to the family's fund. My father worked in construction with Benny for six days a week, while my mother and my sister had jobs in garment factories. Maria was also going to night school to improve her English. Nicholas, Peter, and I were working hard at building a strong base so that we could become self-sufficient blind adults one day.

During the winter months when construction work came to a halt due to bad weather, my father would spend his days sitting by the bedroom window reading repeatedly the code manual for a driver's license. He was eager to gain independence and become the driver for the family. He loved sitting by that window. The bedroom was bright and cozy and looked right out on Beech Street.

In spite of his good intentions to concentrate and study hard, there were always many people passing by eager to engage in a conversation.

He seemed to have no qualms about allowing these interruptions to his tedious and tough study.

"Do you sit by that window because it has good light, or do you sit there just to talk to the neighbors?" my mother would often tease.

By the end of that year my father did receive his driver's licence.

Through word of mouth my parents heard about an apartment house on the market on Van Cortlandt Park Avenue, just one street west of Beech Street.

"It would be our ticket to prosperity if somehow we could buy that house!" my father said to all of us at the dinner table one weekend. "It's an old house that needs lots of work, but work we can do. Little by little while we're collecting rent we can fix up each apartment and soon enough the whole family, married or single, will have a secure place to live in the future."

Without ever seeing the house, I was already planning on how I would arrange my apartment to my liking when I would be old enough to claim it. However my mother quickly ruined my dream with her next comment.

"Yes, it would be nice, but don't get ahead of yourself. You're forgetting the most important thing we need to buy a house," my mother said. "We don't have much savings and the $6,000 bond we had to give to immigration so that our three blind kids could come to America is still tied up for another couple more years. No bank is going to lend us a dime for the down payment, let alone a mortgage. So stop dreaming."

After my relatives had gathered the money to pay the $6,000 bond in 1964, my parents made it their mission to reimburse them as quickly as possible. They did not want to keep their relatives' money tied up for five years. In fact, they had just finished paying the last few hundred dollars remaining from the debt. My mother was right; we now had to wait a couple years for the bond money to be returned to us from the government before we would have any type of down payment for a house.

My mother's three siblings who had immigrated to America years ago were already homeowners. They understood very well that for an immigrant family, home ownership was the most certain road to financial stability. That and hard work. Once they heard about this amazing opportunity, they talked amongst themselves and decided to loan the money back to my parents to be used for the down payment.

We were incredulous when we heard of this kind and generous gesture. It felt so good to have such a loving and supportive family.

I insisted on going with my parents to visit the house and meet with the sellers for the first time. They also were Italian immigrants. The husband and wife and the wife's mother who lived with them, showed us around the property. My parents were happy and felt at ease being able to communicate their thoughts in their native language. To me, it felt like we were visiting more relatives in America whom we hadn't met before.

As we were walking around the ground floor apartment, dreaming of living there soon, my father took a deep breath and said, "You know, this would be the perfect house for my family. There is enough room for everybody, and even enough space for our kids to play music without disturbing the neighbors."

They continued showing us around as much as they could without intruding on the current tenants. Then they invited us to sit at the kitchen table for a cup of coffee. The grandmother reminded me of my Aunt Jenny who lived across from us on Beech Street. She served coffee and some of her homemade cookies, just like Aunt Jenny did every time we visited her. My parents continued chatting about being in America as they shared stories about what they had left behind in Italy.

"Getting back to the house," my father said a one point, "we would like nothing more than to buy this property. We do have the down payment but unfortunately, we haven't been able to find a bank that will lend us money for the mortgage."

The sellers were very gracious and understood our limits. After more friendly conversation with them, we said goodbye, knowing full well a miracle would have to happen for us to own that home.

For the next several days, buying the house was all we talked about. We got together with our relatives every day exploring possibilities, including approaching the owner of a local produce market who was notorious for lending money to Italian immigrants at exorbitant interest rates. Just as we were ready to lose all hope, my parents received a call from the sellers.

"Ever since you visited our place, my wife's mother hasn't stopped talking about how great it would be for your family to live here. We've examined our finances and we think we can carry the loan for the next twenty years. The house is yours if you are still interested."

An explosion of happiness ran through the entire neighborhood once my parents shared the news. And so against all odds, thanks to the benevolence of our extended family and a fellow immigrant, our dream came true. We became homeowners in the spring of 1967, when my parents bought the six-family apartment house at 65 Van Cortlandt Park Avenue in Yonkers, New York.

Our new home was only a block away from Beech Street, but it felt like we had moved far away from a fun family compound. We now had a larger eat-in kitchen, so it was actually easier to invite our relatives to visit us.

Every Sunday featured a big feast. My parents would start early in the morning getting everything ready. My mother would mix the dough for the fresh ravioli and brown the various meats that would simmer for hours in her fresh tomato sauce. My father would work on setting the table. He would bring folding chairs from the basement, where he was already collecting tools and materials that he would use to work on our new house for years to come.

They would have everything under control so they could attend the 9:00 a.m. Mass at the Mount Carmel Church on Park Hill Avenue. They always left the house early enough so they would have plenty of time to chat with any relatives they ran into before the Mass started.

"Ralph already turned the soil in the backyard to plant a garden," my mother would say. "He is planning to install hooks on the ceiling in the basement to hang our fresh sausages to cure during the winter."

"And I'm also planning to build a pergola to grow grapes, so starting next year everybody can come over and sample my Cantisani wine. It will be the best wine in Westchester County, I promise you," my father would add. Lots of laughter followed with congratulations galore.

My parents, along with all the other family members from Basilicata who were homeowners, were trying hard to recreate the same ambiance we all remembered from when we lived on the farm. But this time around, it was all for fun and entertainment, not a matter of survival.

Immediately after church, my mother would come home to tend to her sauce. My father would linger on, chatting with people. Before heading home he would stop at the Café Puglia to buy a copy of *Il Progresso Italo-Americano,* the Italian-language newspaper published daily in New York City. Once home he'd sit at the kitchen table, light a cigarette, and read the paper. Occasionally he would look towards my mother and make a comment about what he was reading. Sooner or later the delicious aroma of the sauce would get to him. He would get out of his chair, grab a fork, and stand next to my mother in front of the stove. He would plunge his fork into the simmering pot, fish out a meatball and pop it into his mouth.

"Ummm," he would exclaim. "These are really good."

"Yes, they're good, but make sure you don't eat too many, or you will ruin your appetite," my mother would admonish. My father would walk back to the table and continue reading. However, it wasn't long before he was back again.

"You are back for more, aren't you?"

"Everything smells so good I can't help myself," he would say.

"If you eat any more meatballs there won't be enough left for anybody else," my mother complained.

"Nonsense," he replied, "I know you, you always make plenty for everybody and then some. It feels good not to have to ration food all the time to make sure we have enough for tomorrow, the next day, and the next after that."

"Yes, it does. It also feels good to be able to go to the store and buy what we want and not just barely what we need."

He would go back to the table and continue reading the Italian newspaper. It was nice to see my parents getting along. They seemed happier than they had been in a long time.

Occasionally my mother would leave the kitchen and come towards our bedrooms and shout, "Are you kids still in bed? Haven't you slept enough? Get out of bed, take a shower, and go to church! You kids need to cleanse your soul. Why don't you animals ever get up and go to church on Sunday?"

"I did cleanse my soul with a few beers last night," Nic would respond. "Isn't that good enough?"

"You are going to go to hell for being such a smart-ass."

My mother would walk away, muttering, "Dear Jesus, how did these kids end up going down this Godless road?"

My sister was the only one of us who complied with church-going. Maria's social circle was composed mainly of Italian immigrants around her age and other single ladies she worked with. She would often meet up with them on Sunday mornings to attend the 11:00 a.m. Mass at Mount Carmel Church. A group of eligible Italian bachelors always waited outside the church. They pretended to be churchgoers, when in reality they were only interested in deciding which young lady they were going to strike up a conversation with after Mass.

Through this type of courtship, my sister met a charming, witty, and handsome Italian immigrant by the name of Tony Dellorso. Everybody in my family was crazy about him. He was like a breath of fresh air. Whenever he came to the house, there was only laughter, laughter, and more laughter. Tony brought along a whole new list of jokes to add to Nic's already large repertoire. Within a year Tony proposed, and preparations for the wedding went into full gear. Every Saturday my mother and my sister would spend the entire day roaming through the shops, exploring everything related to weddings.

With my sister and my mother gone every Saturday, I was the only girl left in the family, so I became the designated Cinderella. I was expected to dust, vacuum, mop, and tidy up the whole house before they came home. One Saturday, I did my work extra quickly and then proceeded to wander through my closet to choose the clothes to take to school with me the following week. Miniskirts had been the rage for some time now and I was beside myself for still not owning one. I pulled out three below-the-knee, double-pleated, wool skirts that I hated wearing because they were so long. I'd had enough of rolling the waistbands to shorten them. I needed to solve this problem somehow.

I held one of the skirts against my body and rolled the hem a few times. *I have an idea!* I ran to the sewing machine, pulled out a pair of scissors, straight pins, a needle, and a spool of thread. I held the spool under a bright lamp. I couldn't actually see the color, but I needed to be sure that the thread was dark enough to match the skirts. Then I went to work.

First I folded the hems of the skirts as many times as I needed to reach the desired length. Then I placed straight pins all along the bottom of the fold to secure it evenly all around. I picked out the stitching of the original hem, and cut off the excess material along the crease.

I had learned how to sew a hem back in Italy when my sister had her sewing business. I used to nag her to show me how to do some stitches. Well, she did, and one of them was the hem stitch. Boy was I happy now! But next came the hard part: threading the needle. Without a threaded needle I could do nothing.

Once again I had an idea. My first instinct was to put the end of the thread in my mouth to wet it. Next I held it horizontally between my lips, tight and straight. With my left hand I held the needle horizontally and glided the eye of the needle between my lips, toward the end of the thread, hoping that with a little luck, it would go in. After a few tries it actually worked. I felt the tip of the thread on the other side of the needle. Bingo!

I grabbed the end of the thread with my teeth and pulled it through. I now had the world by its tail. If my mother had walked in on me and discovered what I was doing, she would have killed me, so I put everything away with a plan to resume the project later that night under the covers. Thankfully, blindness worked to my advantage this time.

When I returned to school on Monday, I brought the three newly shortened skirts with me, along with the cut-off material, making sure not to leave any evidence at home. During the late afternoon off-campus hour, I took the skirts to a dry cleaner located in the same strip of stores where we all used to hang out. On Thursday afternoon I picked them up, and boy was I shocked. They felt brand new—as if they had just come off a department store rack. I was beaming with joy. I walked over to the five-and-dime store with a friend who had more residual vision than me and bought three pairs of fishnet stockings. The store clerk helped me match them to the skirts.

On Friday morning, dressed in one of my newly redesigned skirts I was in vogue and on top of the world, bombarded with compliments from envious friends and even from teachers. I had no idea what my parents' reaction would be when they saw me dressed like that, and to my surprise I couldn't have cared less. I was not willing to give up feeling this good about myself for anybody.

When my mother first saw me as we arrived home late that Friday afternoon, it was anti-climactic. I got no reaction at all. I thought maybe she was winding up for a big explosion, but no such thing happened.

During dinner I was up every chance I got to flaunt my newly fashionable self in front of everybody. I turned myself around with enough speed to cause the pleats of my mini-skirt to flatten against my several inches of exposed thigh, as if to say, "See, there's nothing wrong with this! I just look good, don't I?"

When my mother finally did say something, her tone was loaded with curiosity and maybe even stifled admiration. "Where did you get that skirt, by the way?"

It sure took long enough for her to notice. "What skirt? This skirt?" I asked nonchalantly as if I had been wearing the skirt for months.

"Yes, that skirt."

"They were giving them away at school."

"They were giving them away at school?"

"Yes, they were giving them away at school to girls from families with modest means."

"Really?"

"Yes, really."

Not one other word was uttered. That evening it was clear that we had turned a page. I was deciding for myself how to dress, and my mother could no longer control me.

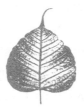

CHAPTER 82

JULIEN

Nicholas and I were well into our teens by now and like most teenagers, our heads were filled with romantic daydreams. In our house of course, the topic of boyfriends and girlfriends was clearly off the table. We blind kids were not allowed to think about or become engaged in such activities until we were done with our studies and ready to embark on our careers. But this rule was mainly aimed at me because I was the girl and also the most likely suspect to mess up somehow.

The beginning of every school year came with the usual lectures and advice from my parents. "Buckle down! Don't get in trouble! Don't make friends with people who will take you down the wrong path!" I had calluses in my ears from hearing that over and over. "At your age it is too distracting to get involved with girlfriends or boyfriends," my parents would take turns telling us.

In spite of their concerns, my parents were too busy trying to make a living to ever come to the school during the week and monitor how we spent our free time. On weekends I had an understanding with my male friends that if they phoned me and I wasn't the one answering the phone, they would simply ask to speak to Nic. And for a long time, it worked like a charm.

In the spring, a boy name Julien asked me to go to the movies with him after school on a Friday afternoon. I liked him so I accepted the invitation; but now I had to come up with an excuse for staying at school late. I was still on the cheerleading team and on occasion I did spend part of the weekend at the residential school with the cheerleading squad practicing before a big tournament.

I decided to tell my parents I had cheerleading practice that Friday afternoon and would take the subway home to 242nd Street with Nic, who was also staying late to practice with his wrestling team. None of this was true, of course, but Nic agreed to meet me at the 242nd Street train station at 6:00 p.m. We would then call our father to come pick us up. My parents accepted the plan. It seemed foolproof. After all Nic had done it a number of times before with his wrestling practice, so there were no suspicious questions asked.

So on Friday afternoon, I told the school bus driver I wouldn't be riding home due to an after-school activity. After the movie, Julien and I made sure that by 6:00 p.m., we were at the 242nd Street subway station waiting to meet Nic as prearranged. Julien was legally blind, but he had enough vision to read small print and was able to recognize people from a distance. Calm and collected we waited for Nic for at least thirty minutes. There was no Nic in sight.

We then began thinking that maybe he had misunderstood the address of the station and was waiting for us at the 238th Street station. We rode back to 238th Street and started shouting his name up and down the platform and around the nearby streets. Failing to find Nic, we returned to the original meeting point.

It was well after 7 o'clock now and we began to panic. It was getting dark but luckily the lighting didn't affect Julien's vision, but it certainly hampered mine. I couldn't see anything. Our foolproof plan was falling apart. My stomach tightened and my mouth started drying up. We continued to shout Nic's name around the station without any luck. Finally, Julien decided to call my house and ask to speak to Nic. We located a phone booth and luckily Julien had the right change in his pockets to insert into the pay phone.

My father answered the call. "Hello?"

"Hello, Mr. Cantisani, may I speak to Nic, please?"

"Nic? Nic no home. Who is you?" my father asked him.

"I'm John, a friend. Can I speak to Nic?"

"Nic no home," my father repeated with a gruff tone and hung up.

Julien was quiet. He then started apologizing for what was happening. "He's not home, so where in the hell is he?"

"He's somewhere waiting for us," I said.

Another hour went by as we raced from one station to the other, shouting Nic's name to no avail.

We located another phone booth and Julien called my house again. This time Nic answered.

"Nic, where in the hell were you???" Julien said.

"I waited and waited for you at the 242nd Street station, but for some reason we missed each other so I had to come home and tell mom and dad that I couldn't find you guys," said Nic. "I didn't know what else to tell them so they called the school and reported Carmela missing."

I nearly fainted. And there it was; we knew the cat was out of the bag and all hell was coming our way . . .

"So what do we do now?" asked Julien.

"Take Carmela back to school and I'll tell dad to pick her up at the back gate."

Riding the subway back to 238th Street and then walking two blocks to Pelham Parkway and the back gate of the school was torture, torture, torture. Nothing had prepared me for this.

Once we got to the school's back gate, Julien insisted on waiting with me.

"No, you really shouldn't because it will just add fuel to the fire if my father sees you with me."

Julien kissed me and said, "I'll be hiding behind these bushes to make sure you are safe until your dad picks you up. Your father better not lay a hand on you!"

I stood waiting about ten feet from the two lamp posts dotting the edges of the school's back gate. Thick foliage from the trees towering over me darkened the night. I waited in fear wondering what kind of punishment was in store for me.

Every car that drove by, even though it didn't slow down, sounded to me like hell was coming. When my father finally arrived, he drove so slowly it sounded as if a hearse were pulling in. I felt queasy. He pulled up in front of me. I opened the passenger door and got in the car without exchanging a word with him. We rode home in total silence. Having spent a few years as a prisoner of war in World War II, he had learned how to choose his battles and to avoid futile talk.

When I walked into the house there was complete silence as though a dead body was being rolled into the room. I knew that the longer my mother waited before she exploded, the fiercer she would be when she finally did. I decided that no matter what comment or accusation they would throw at me, I was not going to gratify anyone with a reaction.

"You're suspended from school until further notice!" my mother finally barked in my face. "Are you happy, now?" Her voice screeched through her teeth like the tires of a big truck trying to stop before a huge crash. The name-calling, false accusations, and menacing threats went on and on, but I held onto my precious vow of silence and she hated it. She was expecting a volatile reaction from me that would give her a good excuse to strike me and find some release to her anger, but I stood strong. The weekend went by without my speaking a single word to my parents.

On Monday morning I stayed in bed, since I was suspended from school. My father and my sister left for work, Nic and Peter left for school, and shortly thereafter my mother left the house dressed as though as she was going to take care of some official business. I was happy to be home alone. Here was my chance to call Julien to find out whether he had been suspended as well, and if so, for how long.

When I picked up the receiver, I realized that a lock had been installed on the rotary dial of the phone. *How dare they do that?!* I felt as though a heavy metal cage had surrounded my body. I was stunned, angry, and hated my parents for isolating me in this way. I stood immobile, holding the receiver to my ear, just listening to the dial tone in disbelief, not knowing what to do next. Suddenly a friendly voice interrupted the awful sound, saying, "Operator, may I help you?" My heart warmed.

"Operator," I said, "I'm blind and I need help placing a call."

"Sure," she replied. I gave her the number and was immediately connected with Julien.

Our conversation was brief because I didn't want to get caught speaking on the phone. Julien told me he had been suspended as well, but for how long he didn't know.

My mother was gone all morning; much longer than I expected. About noon, she came home but she was not alone. She had gone somewhere with her sister Jenny and her brother Dominic and his wife Mary. Wow, I thought to myself, where have they been? My Uncle Dominic took a day off work at ConEdison to go somewhere with my mother? This was a real family crisis and my mother's siblings had come to her rescue. My mother ordered me to sit at the table and eat lunch with them. We ate mostly in silence. After lunch, while they all sipped *anisette*-spiked espresso, I finally learned my fate.

"We went to speak to the school's principal," shouted my mother. "He says you are only allowed to go back to school if we take you to see a doctor and he examines you to make sure that nothing happened between you and that boy!"

I knew that meant the school principal thought I had had sex with Julien. It seemed my family suspected the same thing. I could not believe my ears.

"What do you have? Dust in your head?" shouted my uncle. "Your parents made a lot of sacrifices to give you a good life and this is how you're paying them back?" he continued. Why were my relatives, who had been so very nice to me suddenly turning on me like this? I hadn't done anything wrong except lying about my whereabouts, and all of a sudden everybody was jumping to conclusions. No one had bothered to ask me what Julien and I had done that previous Friday afternoon. They were simply making assumptions based on no information. My relatives and my mother took turns reprimanding me.

I hated them all. When would this torture end? Yeah sure, I thought to myself, I'm guilty, all right. Everything is my fault. It's also my fault the school principal is a male chauvinist bastard and pathetically jealous of my youth. Seething with anger, I nevertheless managed to keep my mouth shut. The ordeal ended when they all went home and I was able to return to my room to find some peace and solitude.

On Thursday evening my parents took me to our Italian family doctor who had after-dinner visiting hours. They presented the note from the school requesting proof of my virginity. He agreed to examine me.

After a long, grueling week of waiting for each painful second to pass, my suspension was finally over. On Monday morning as I was getting ready to leave for school for the week, my mother snatched her last opportunity to fill my head with admonitions. "You better keep your nose out of trouble," she said with conviction. "This is the last chance you have. If I hear that you even get near that boy one more time, I'll send you to a school run by nuns!"

"Yeah, yeah, yeah," I said angrily. "You send me to the nuns and I will bring home a report card full of F's, and then we'll see who wins!"

"We'll see about that!" she retorted.

With the doctor's letter in hand I returned to school dressed in dark, conservative clothing to better blend in with the furniture and the walls. I was ashamed and wanted to hide my very existence, not knowing who knew what, and which version of the story they had heard. Who is on my side, I wondered.

As I stood in line waiting to file into the assembly hall, three female teachers approached me. They put their arms around me and said, "Welcome back. We are very sorry and angry that you had to go through that awful experience." They took turns holding me with tears in their eyes. That warm gesture gave me the confidence I needed so that I could breathe easily again.

Sometime later I learned each of those teachers had spent two years as a volunteer in the Peace Corps in some far-off part of the world. Now all three of them were active in the women's liberation movement, where they were fighting to change the very same antiquated and chauvinistic practices I had just experienced.

Throughout the day, I was pleasantly surprised at the warm and supportive reception I received from everyone around the school. Once I finally met up with Julien during the lunch hour, he apologized again for the ordeal and for being allowed to return to school after just one day of suspension. He then presented me with a gift his mother had helped him buy: a beautiful, heavy, gold locket with a diamond in the middle of a heart-shaped face.

"No thank-yous are necessary," he said. "I just want you to have it and I thank you for being you!"

Julien and I remained friends and continued to socialize. The teachers reassured us that they would profess ignorance if my parents ever asked about us. I kept that locket for many, many years, until it was stolen from me during a trip to Morocco.

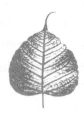

CHAPTER 83

THE COURAGE TO DREAM BIG DREAMS

During my junior year, I had to choose a major so that the teacher of that subject could become my advisor and help me with my post–high school plans. I picked French by default. I did very well in the class, I liked the teacher, and I couldn't think of any other subject I enjoyed enough to select as a major. Languages came naturally to me, and I had always been intrigued by careers that involved languages and travel.

The next subject in line would have been music, but that was a life-long, complicated story. Thanks to my current piano teachers, I had improved my playing significantly, but classical music as a career-choice was an old story that I had put to rest during middle school back in Italy. I knew in my heart what my fears were and I was not willing to revisit them. I was simply not disciplined enough to pursue a career that required so much commitment and dedication.

I had been performing at school recitals at the end of every year since 9th grade. To prepare for the junior year recital, my teacher had given me a few choices for the piece I could learn and perform. She played all of them for me before I made my selection. I liked all of the pieces, but when I heard her play the *Scherzo* No. 2 in B flat minor by Frédéric Chopin, I fell in love with it immediately.

"This piece is technically demanding, but with your passion, I really think you can pull it off," she said.

"It sounds so difficult! Are you sure I can do it?"

"Yes, I'm sure. You will make me proud."

When she handed me the folder containing the Braille sheet music I couldn't believe how thick it was. It felt like it contained all the pieces I had ever learned in my life (and then some). *I don't care how complex and challenging it is, I'm going to learn it and perform it perfectly.*

"You're going to make me proud. I'm counting on you," she said as she patted me on the shoulder. It felt good to have someone believe in me. I wasted no time getting started. I was so mesmerized by this musical composition that I even took the music home with me every weekend to maximize my progress.

The Chopin piece consumed me. Playing the piece always made me feel liberated. It validated my own emotions — at times tumultuous, and at other times soft and romantic. This was a characteristic for which I often received criticism, but there it was in Chopin's music. As I committed the piece to memory some of my favorite passages would stream through my head over and over, even when I wasn't playing them, bringing a sense of fulfillment and confidence I had never felt before. By April of 1968, one month before the piano recital, I had my performance number under control.

One day near the end of my piano practice hour, just before the morning recess, I sensed a presence, as though someone were looking through the glass door watching me play. When the bell rang, I took my music and headed out the door. The presence of my French teacher was unmistakable; I'd recognize his distinguished and expensive cologne anywhere.

"*Bonjour Mademoiselle,*" he said with his usual French flair.

"*Bonjour Monsieur,*" I replied shyly.

"Beautiful, beautiful playing," he said. "Congratulations! I'm looking forward to attending your recital."

"*Merci Monsieur,*" I answered, blushing.

"I need to talk to you as your advisor. Is this a good time?"

"Of course," I said.

We would occasionally meet in his classroom during the morning break for one reason or another. I was secretly pleased and happy whenever one of these spontaneous rendezvous occurred. Together we walked to his classroom, which happened to be on the same floor as the music rooms. He closed the door behind him gently, placed his left palm onto the small of my back and guided me to the swivel chair by his desk. Once I was seated he glided behind me, brushing against my waist-length hair giving me butterflies.

He leaned against the open window about three feet away from me before saying anything. I focused on shapes of sunlight cast on the wall across from me as I avoided looking in his direction. It was interesting how tricky the progression of my eye disease could be. Depending upon how the sun illuminated a room, at times I felt as though I could see quite a bit. On this particular day the lighting was perfect. Knowing where everything was in his classroom, I could act as sighted as I wanted and not risk appearing foolish by focusing on the wrong thing. I finally turned my gaze toward my French teacher.

"I know there is still plenty of time left before you have to make the final decision as to what you want to do with your future, but as your advisor I want to make sure that I guide you in the right direction. Have you had a chance to think more about your options?" he asked.

An ensemble of mixed emotions roared through me at the sound of his words. I placed my right elbow on his desk and leaned on my folded fingers, thinking about how I could avoid discussing this topic.

"Well, I really don't know. Every time I try to think about my options, everything seems so confusing and complicated."

"I know, but let's try to narrow things down," he said. "Is there anything that you see yourself doing and being happy doing?"

"I found the visit to the United Nations last month with the French Club very intriguing. I would be very happy to be in that kind of ambiance forever. Maybe I should become an interpreter. Is that a hard thing to do?" *Was that a stupid thing to say? Why doesn't he just tell me what to do?*

A long pause followed. "No, being an interpreter would not be a hard thing for you to do. Learning languages for you, comes naturally, and that's a big hurdle right there," he said after a long exhalation. "But, are you aware of the daily ins and outs of the work?"

"No, not really. I know that you interpret from one language to another. I think it's a job without much fuss, and most of it is done orally which would be great for me," I replied.

"Without much fuss? I'm not sure about that. It pays well, and initially it can be very interesting and exciting. You're often meeting new people from all parts of the world, which you would like, of course. There is usually some travel involved, which you would also like. But make sure you aren't hijacked by the glamorous appearance of the job. You have to be current on a wide range of topics which means you have to read constantly. But the biggest drawback is that interpreters spend most of their time confined to a booth interpreting from one language to another though headphones and a microphone without adding or subtracting even a smidgeon of their personal thoughts. I could be wrong, but you seem too feisty and creative to tolerate the monotony and constraints of that job."

Well, now I really don't know what I want to do. Being confined to an interpreting booth sounds as bad as being confined to a piano bench practicing scales and arpeggios to the beat of a metronome for hours on end.

"Interpreting doesn't begin and end at the United Nations, you know. You could also work as a court interpreter or a medical interpreter," he added.

No matter what we talked about, I never got tired of spending time with my French teacher. He was so smart, knowledgeable, confident, and worldly. I hoped I could be just like him one day.

Yes, he's right, I am feisty and creative, with a charming personality, which should push me right along, but how much of this will really matter in the turmoil of approaching a whole new life? Like most teenagers, I had difficulty being frank about my short-comings, and I didn't want to divulge, particularly to him, any weaknesses or the insecurities I felt.

I do well in French and piano class because I like these subjects, and they come naturally to me. But when I have to read Shakespeare, I'm at a total loss. I feel like there are gaps in my knowledge. I don't have a strong base in all the subjects at American schools like I did in Italy. I don't know how I can be successful in any field with all these gaps.

"OK," I said, "If it's not interpreting, then maybe I can work in an airport. That might take care of my wanderlust."

"And what would you do at the airport?" he asked.

"Oh, I don't know. Maybe I can announce flights in different languages, or better yet I can be an air traffic controller. I would be in seventh Heaven doing that job. It's the kind of job that would give you a lot of adrenaline."

He immediately broke into a very amused laugher. "Wow, that sounds more like you. Tossing around the impossible is one way to identify what IS possible. You are the most intriguing person I have ever met in my life. You have the courage to dream big dreams and that will take you far," he said reassuringly.

"I've had a chance to talk with your piano teacher a few times," he said with a more serious tone. "She is amazed at how much your piano playing has improved. She would like you to consider going to music school and I agree. It would be a shame for you to waste such a talent. Perhaps we can explore the possibilities of turning it into a career. You are emotionally rich, you have a lot to offer to the world, and you shouldn't hold back."

His words sounded a familiar note in my head — a note that triggered a knot of sadness in my throat. I struggled to swallow. No, I'm not emotionally rich, I thought. I'm emotionally fragile and that's the problem. Of course I enjoy playing the piano and I love classical music, but I feel like such a fraud because I don't like anything else connected with classical music. The reason I play so well is that I get to choose the pieces that I want to learn. Other than having to forgo my long nails, I don't have many restrictions with my current teacher. However, a career in music requires a much bigger commitment than just learning to play pieces that you like. It requires constant practice and a dedication to classical music; music I don't want to play full time.

Perhaps the reason I could not make music a career at this point could be traced back to my music teacher in elementary school in Italy. She stifled the natural talent I was lucky to have and made it very painful for me to develop my full potential. My grade school piano teacher didn't know how to teach children like me. She thought the harder she pushed, the better the results would be. In my case it worked the other way around.

Will there ever be anything I can do well enough to make it a career? I wonder what my life will look like in the future. What kind of work will I be doing? Will I have a family of my own? Will I have made the right choices? And most importantly, will I be happy?

"I love to watch you think," my French teacher said softly, interrupting my trance. "You have beautiful eyes and they are very expressive," he added with the captivating allure only a Frenchman possesses. The room was filled with fresh morning air, heavily scented with spring aromas. I turned my gaze toward the open window in an effort to mask the stirred-up emotions created by the power of flattery.

My favorite passage from the Chopin *Scherzo* started flowing through my head like a long stream of warm, magical light as I gently drifted into another world. I felt transported far, far away, escorted on the wings of a thousand birds as though I were floating through long curtains of times lapsed, dusty wine grapes in a wicker basket … a streak of red filament … an old empty train …

CHAPTER 84

FACING REALITY

Only a few days had passed since my father's funeral in early January 1999. I was still in New York grieving his loss with my mother. Time passing had taken on a life of its own. It would take hours for one minute to pass, or we could spend hours reminiscing and it seemed like only minutes had gone by. My father's death was a harsh reminder that time with our loved ones is precious.

I thought with nostalgia, of my teenage years when I could take my parents for granted. It was also a time when I thought naively if I stared at the moon long enough, it would carry my romantic thoughts to a special someone. I wished that I could return to that dream world instead of living in the painful present. Suddenly the jarring ring of the telephone jolted me to my feet. By the second ring I answered and recognized my sister's voice on the other end of the call.

"What are you guys doing? Are you day-dreaming? Aren't you hungry?" my sister asked, calling from her kitchen upstairs. "It's after 12 o'clock. Lunch is ready. Bring mom upstairs."

"We'll be right up," I replied, and hung up the phone.

During lunch, Maria informed us that she and her husband Tony were going to return to Florida for a few days to finish the repairs in their water-damaged vacation home. With my father's sudden passing they had returned to New York in a hurry before the work was complete.

"I wish Benny had called us sooner to tell us how sick dad was. I don't understand why he waited so long. We could have come back from Florida a lot sooner. At least I would have had a chance to say goodbye before he died," my sister said.

"I called from California every day to check on dad, but either Benny wasn't really aware of his failing condition or he was in denial.

I would have jumped on a plane immediately if I had thought the end might be near. So I didn't get to say goodbye to dad, either. Don't worry. Just do what you have to do. I'll be here with mom," I said, reassuring my sister.

Maria's youngest children, Frank and Rosie, had finished college and were gainfully employed. But being good Italian kids, still lived at home so they could save money for a more financially stable future. While my sister and her husband were gone, it was nice to have dinner most nights with my niece, nephew, and my mother. With a smaller group, dinner conversations can be more intimate. My mornings though, for the rest of the month of January, I spent reminiscing and exchanging stories with my mother, hoping it would help both of us grieve and deal with the loss of my father.

Ever since I had noticed the first symptoms of Alzheimer's in my mother's behavior, I had been researching the disease. As I spent more time with her, I had been thus far successful in helping her coast through her daily routine without any big hurdles. If she seemed to be headed toward a negative plunge, I would redirect her train of thought. I filled in the gaps when she experienced a memory blank, and helped her accomplish certain tasks that she was now finding frustrating and difficult.

With this type of low-key support, she remained highly functional, fairly happy, and hardly aware she was suffering from this devastating disease.

One evening while the four of us were having dinner, my niece Rosie suggested, "Why don't you tell Nonna Rosa the story about the passenger on the plane who complained about sitting next to your guide dog?"

"You want me to tell her about that?" I said.

"Yes, she'll get a kick out of it. I want to see her laugh!"

"So ma, listen to this story: One time after visiting you guys, I boarded a plane at JFK bound for San Francisco. This was before the mileage plus programs started, so Business Class was pretty much always empty. I was seated in the middle seat in bulkhead with my guide dog, McCloud, lying on the floor on my right. Do you all remember McCloud?"

"Oh, I remember McCloud. You brought him to my class one time when I was in grade school," my niece said nostalgically.

"Yes, I remember that, too. Your classmates were all so cute and asked so many questions about how guide dogs work. That was a fun day," I said, and continued with the story.

"The window seat was left empty to give the dog extra room, and a gentleman occupied the aisle seat on my left. In those days if you complained about something, more often than not you landed in one of those big, comfortable seats in Business Class. When the flight attendant walked by, the gentleman on my left asked her, 'Can I be moved to a different seat? I didn't know that I was going to be seated next to a dog.'

She looked at him and said, 'Sir, the plane is full but let me see what I can do.'

I immediately looked up at her and said, 'By all means, ma'am, do find him a different seat because I had no idea that I was going to be seated next to an asshole.'"

My mother immediately burst out laughing, "You said that? In front of everybody?"

"Yes I did."

"Well, with your sharp tongue, I wouldn't put it past you," my mother commented.

"Almost immediately the gentleman sitting directly behind me in the middle seat stood up and volunteered to switch seats. Well, after the asshole moved, he was no longer sitting next to a dog. Instead, he was tightly wedged between two passengers and had the back of my fully reclined seat in his face, with no room in front of him to stretch his legs. Well, the moral of the story," I told my mother, "is if you're sitting next to a dog, before you complain, make sure you're not sitting next to a real bitch like me."

Laughter, laughter, laughter in all directions. Then my mother said, "How can you have your answers always ready like that?"

"I don't know" I replied, "I must have learned it from you!"

"No you didn't! I never had snappy answers ready like that. You couldn't have learned it from me. I'm not that feisty!"

"Yes you are," I said. "I heard you lots of times arguing with dad with snappy answers ready."

Before I even finished saying that, I realized it was the wrong topic to raise. A long pause followed. She leaned forward and put her left elbow on the table, placed her chin in the palm of her hand, and said in a solemn tone, "Well, your father was not an easy man to get along with." A deep sigh followed. "Remember, if it weren't for women who always sacrifice everything to keep their families together, the world would have gone down the toilet a long time ago," she said resignedly.

"I know," I replied, and gently redirected the topic. "Do you remember when we went gambling at Lake Tahoe and Peter and I kept stealing your winnings from you?"

"Of course I remember," she said, with a happier tone and a giggle. "You guys lost all of your money and then you stole from me so that you could play some more."

"You almost agreed to come skiing with us the next day, remember?"

"No, I didn't. Now you're lying! But your father and I enjoyed watching you ski. We had never seen that before. I think you were training for that big race where you won gold medals, weren't you?"

"Yes, in fact that was New Year's Day of 1985, and I was beginning to train for the World Championships of 1986, that were going to be held in Sweden."

"Wow, that was a long time ago!" my mother exclaimed.

"Time flies," I added.

"We all know that you did three international competitions and lots of racing before that, but sadly, we've never had a chance to really talk about it much. This is a perfect time for you to tell us all about it," said Rosie.

"Yeah," added my nephew Frank. "It's nice and snowy outside. We can roast some chestnuts and talk about skiing all night. When did you start skiing, anyway?"

Wow, I was actually flattered that my niece and nephew were interested enough to hear the details of my skiing. I had spent years trying to get them to share the sport with me, but for some reason it had never worked out. Rosie was the only member of my large family who ever managed to come out to California to ski with me. Well, I thought to myself, if they really want to hear it this is as good a time as any to share the stories about my ski competitions.

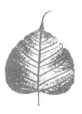

CHAPTER 85

GOING FOR THE GOLD, 1986

I gave skiing a go for the first time in the mid-70s when the sport was just starting to become available to blind people. A series of races in the years that followed landed me on the U.S. Disabled Ski Team in 1985. Being on the this team qualified me to compete in the 1986 World Championship for the Disabled.

Cliff May, an avid skier and passionate racer who lived at the ski resort in Kirkwood, California, became my official ski guide for racing. We trained hard every chance we had to prepare for the world competition in April of 1986, in Salen, Sweden, and felt confident we had a good chance to win.

The blind competitors were divided into three categories. The B-1 Category was for skiers who had no functional vision at all, except perhaps for light perception. The B-2 Category was for skiers who could see only the distance of one gate at a time in front of them on the racecourse. B-3 Category competitors had enough vision to see several gates at a time and had no trouble seeing their ski guide in front of them.

Within these categories, it was sometimes difficult to draw the line between a B-2 or a B-3 skier. For the most part, there were no doubts about who was a B-1 skier. Having only light perception, I landed a spot in the Blind Women's Division in the B-1 Category.

The more I got into the story with my nephew and niece, the more excited I became. It was like I was reliving the experience. I could hear and visualize all the details. We were in Salen, Sweden, for two weeks to compete in the World Championships. The first race scheduled was the downhill, on April 13, 1986.

"Wow!" exclaimed my ski guide, Cliff May, as he looked down on the ski slope. "It looks like they did a good job grooming the racecourse.

The few inches of snow we got last night really helped. At least we won't have to deal with the awful icy conditions we've been struggling with all week. I think we have perfect conditions to win this race ... Are you awake? Did you hear what I said?"

"Yes, I'm awake and ready; don't worry," I said. I sighed deeply to settle my nerves. "We'll be unloading the chairlift soon. We're just about to pass the last ski tower," Cliff warned me.

My stomach went queasy. Cliff always sounded calm and collected. I guess we both did a pretty good job not showing signs of anxiety or lack of confidence before a race.

"We're just about there," he said. "You already know what we are going to do when we get off the lift, but I'll tell you anyway. As soon as we unload, we'll ski straight out for about 10 feet and then we'll make an easy left turn, followed by a stop."

As we approached the unloading deck, the lift operator saw the orange bib with large black letters that read Blind Racer, and signaled to Cliff to determine if he should slow down the lift. Cliff shouted, "No need to slow it down."

"OK. Here we go. Let's scoot forward, tips up, 3 ... 2 ... 1 ... stand, go ... keep going straight, go ... go ... go ... tips gently to the left, go ... go ... and left to a stop."

Once we had stopped, Cliff told me, "We're not too far from where the team is starting to line up. Let's not waste any energy before the race. Just grab my pole and let's ski down there together."

Once in line with my category, I heard the sound of footsteps behind me and felt a sudden rub on my shoulders. It was our coach, Bob Webber. He leaned down and whispered in my ear, "You're gonna do just fine. You and Cliff have trained hard and it really shows." He turned to Cliff and said, "You guys need to move up to the front quickly. As you know the women's B-1 category is going down first and the race is starting soon." Then he shook Cliff's hand, slapped him on the shoulder, said, "Good luck, you two," and he was gone.

Our coach's words of encouragement provided a welcome break from the sick feeling I had been dragging along with me since I had awakened that morning. But as soon as Cliff gave me the command to glide forward, the sick feeling quickly returned. The closer we got to the starting gate, the worse I felt.

We slowly inched our way into the starting gate. Cliff carefully positioned my ski poles into the right spot making absolutely sure not to touch the timing wand. My knees were perfectly bent, my skis in perfect alignment, and my nerves in perfect shambles.

"We'll do the run exactly the way we did the last four practice runs, OK?" Cliff said.

"OK," I replied, sounding far more confident than I felt.

It was not the first time I'd heard Cliff's instructions. We'd gone over these details at least a dozen times. But it was good to hear them again at the last possible moment.

"I will give you the starting command like we've always done: three, two, one, go. I will take off on the 'one,' and you, right behind me on the 'go.' That way, you'll be just behind me in perfect sync. For the first two gates we'll keep our skis in a gentle snowplow, just to control our speed on the steep part. As soon as I call 'number one,' put your skis in a parallel position so we can gain some speed. Don't worry; it's going to be a piece of cake. We know what we're doing!"

Suddenly I felt the urge to pee, and as if I was going to tremble into total uselessness. *This feels like torture.* I felt like I was waiting in line for a guillotine to chop off my head. I had experienced stage fright before, but not like this. *How in the Hell am I going to pull this off? I have to win this race, but if I don't, it feels like my life will be over! How in the world did I get here anyway?*

"Once I start the timer, you have 5 seconds to start," announced the starting gatekeeper. "Are you ready?"

My stomach convulsed. To avoid vomiting, my mind flashed thousands of miles away and back at least a decade, to January of 1976.

One afternoon my blind roommate, JJ, asked me if I wanted to go skiing the upcoming weekend.

"How did you come up with that?" I asked.

"It's organized through the adaptive Physical Education program at Monterey Peninsula College. It's only $25, and it includes door-to-door transportation to the ski resort up in Lake Tahoe. What do you think?"

"Hell, yeah!" I exclaimed, "$25 is a deal for us unemployed college graduates. Somebody must really want us to go skiing!"

"Apparently it's a group of guys who lost a limb or two in Vietnam. They formed an organization called The National Handicapped Sportsmen Something-or-other and they want to experiment with different techniques in teaching and guiding blind people on the ski slopes. We're gonna be guinea pigs!" JJ shouted happily.

"Sounds great to me, especially the 'bunch of guys' part. Do we get to Braille them as part of the experiment?" I asked.

"All right you smart bitch, don't go embarrassing me. Nobody wants you anyway. You're blind and you're a smart ass," she reprimanded.

"Well, nobody wants you either, because you're blind and smart," I replied.

"Yeah, yeah, I know. The dating scene for blind women sucks sometimes, but you better behave, otherwise one of those handsome ski instructors is gonna leave you stranded on top of a hill and then you'll have to depend on a coyote to guide you down to the bottom if you're lucky," said JJ, laughing.

"Kind of like that ex-boyfriend of yours, who left you stranded in a bar in Amsterdam, remember?" JJ continued. "Tell me again what happened?"

"Oh, are we elaborating on past experiences, is that it?" I asked JJ.

"Why not? It feels good to vent about this stuff once in a while!" JJ replied, taking something out of the cupboard. "How about a rum and Coke?" she suggested.

"Yuck, no, you know I don't like rum and Coke."

"Then mix your own damn martini," she said.

"Isn't it kind of early for a drink? It's not even dark out yet," I said, looking toward the window.

"Maybe for you it's not dark," responded JJ. "For me it's dark all the time, so I can drink whenever I want."

"Ha, ha, ha, who's being the smart-ass now?" I laughed.

"Get yourself a martini, will you? You are so much easier to deal with when you are under the influence. So let's hear it; why did he leave you stranded in the bar anyway?" JJ asked.

"Oh, because he got pissed off about something and didn't have the balls to stay for the argument. Being stranded in a bar wouldn't have been so bad, except I didn't remember the name of the hotel where we were staying, and I didn't have my passport on me, so getting back to our hotel would have been a real problem. Luckily, the asshole came back for me before the bar closed, but until he showed up I was sick with anxiety about what I would do in case the son-of-a-bitch didn't come back."

"Was he short?" JJ asked.

"Yeah, why?"

"Oh, poor baby," exclaimed JJ. "He needed to corner a blind woman into an impossible situation just to see how tall he could feel. What a loser. But I bet that taught you not to break the cardinal rule. Don't ever walk out the door without being prepared to cover your own blind ass no matter what," JJ chastised.

"Oh, stop being so philosophical, we're allowed to make mistakes, aren't we?" I asked. "After all, we're not professionals at being blind; we're just regular humans, with feelings like everyone else."

"Yeah, I know, you're right," JJ responded. "But you know what, though? All jokes aside, no matter which incident we talk about, nothing tops the theater experience you had when the director wouldn't even let you audition to play the blind woman in 'Wait Until Dark.'"

"Oh, I absolutely agree. That was awful," I said.

"If that's not the most quintessential form of blatant discrimination, I don't know what is," JJ said.

"Yeah, I agree; especially when she said, 'A lot of unexpected things can happen on stage. It would be too risky for a blind person.'"

"Didn't the idiot know that the set-up on stage is quite easy for a blind person to memorize because we're used to navigating in the dark? That makes it actually safer for a blind person than a sighted person to play that role — especially in the dark!" JJ said.

"Yeah; you know that, and I know that, but she didn't know that, and she was in charge. But, as you know, real poetic justice was served on a silver platter in that case for sure," I said.

"Yeah, two performances into the run the actress they chose to play the role of the blind woman tripped while trying to navigate in the dark and broke her leg. They had to cancel the rest of the performances as a result. Wasn't that sweet?"

As two unemployed blind college graduates living on $275 a month of Social Security Income, ski weekends were not a recreational option for us unless they were practically free, and this one most certainly was. JJ made the arrangements.

As unprepared for cold weather as one could possibly be, the following Friday afternoon we walked a few hundred yards from our apartment to the designated area at the junior college campus. Someone picked us up in a golf cart to take us to the departure spot. On the way the driver made a sharp turn to the left, sending me sliding off the cart into the bushes.

"We just lost Carmela!" JJ shouted in her pronounced Southern drawl. She broke into the most full-throated hilarious laughter imaginable. Even the crows seemed to partake in the festivities, cawing loudly. The driver was horrified.

"Are you all right?" she asked.

"Losing a blind passenger is worth a lot of points, you know, if you're keeping score with other drivers," JJ told the driver.

Once at the ski resort, the accommodations were very basic. During the night I had to thaw out my feet in hot water several times. I was definitely not prepared for such cold weather.

The next morning after breakfast, we stood in line for rental equipment. My ski instructor showed me what ski boots look like and how to put them on. He then showed me what skis look like and how the bindings work. Then he showed me how to walk in ski boots safely, so that I wouldn't slip and fall down the stairs.

Once outside, he helped me put my skis on. He showed me how to glide my skis back and forth, how to sidestep, how to use ski poles for both balance and to help remain stationary on the snow. We practiced for quite a while until he thought I was ready to learn how to snowplow.

"Glide forward and push your tails out and your ski edges in as though you were shaping a slice of pizza." After a few tries, he said, "You're a natural! Just so you know, you can learn to ski just like sighted people. The only difference is that you can't do it alone. You will need to ski with a well-trained guide in front of you who can give you accurate verbal commands so that you can move down the mountain safely. The first thing we're going to do, though, is to make sure that you respond to the most important and crucial command in the sport. When I give the command 'sit!' you must sit on the snow immediately, no matter what you're doing because it means that danger is imminent. Before we move forward from here, you have to demonstrate that you can respond to that command immediately; otherwise, you will not be allowed to ski. Are you ready to try?" he asked.

"Yes, of course," I responded.

"Let's practice. I'm going to move away from you about 10 feet. I will tell you to glide forward, and when I call 'sit!' you must sit immediately. Ready?" he said. "Glide forward! Keep coming ... forward ... forward ... forward ... good! Forward ... sit!"

Unfortunately I was so enthralled with the sensation of gliding, moving, and gaining speed that I forgot to sit and so, a few feet later, I found myself skiing straight into my ski instructor's arms.

"Is this what you call imminent danger?" I asked.

"Don't be a smart-ass. If I had been a tree you would not be laughing right now. Let's try it again!"

Yes, that's how my first ski experience started about a decade ago, with lots of laughter and lots of fun. And now I was on the verge of throwing up at the starting gate of a world competition.

The time keeper repeated, "You have five seconds. Skier ready?"

"Yes, I'm ready" I responded. I heard the first beep and Cliff started the commands.

As planned, and as we had done many, many times before in practice runs, I pushed out the starting gate on the "go" command. I felt the timing wand brush against my right leg and, thanks to our meticulous planning in practice, I ended up right behind Cliff in perfect sync.

We cruised through the first two turns perfectly, which was just what I needed to gain confidence and shake off stage fright. I felt like a racehorse, ready to fly through every gate without incident and get through the finish line, clocking our best time ever.

Much to my surprise, after we went around the third gate successfully, Cliff called a "tuck" command with a higher tone in his voice. "Tuck … tuck … tuck … tuck!" he shouted confidently. *What in the hell is he doing? This was not part of the plan! This is so risky!* I was petrified. We were moving so fast I thought for sure I was going to lose control at any moment. I knew that I had to follow him at all costs, because there was no way that I could communicate to him to slow down.

But what scared me was the fact that in the tuck position, I could gain way too much speed, possibly ski onto his tails, knock both of us off balance, and create the most spectacular aerobatic blowout ever, completely obliterating our chances of winning. I got myself into a partial tuck position, which made me feel awkward. I felt as though I were getting ready to take a dump, rather than skiing gracefully in a world competition.

After a couple more turns in a partial tuck position, the tone of Cliff's voice changed, and so did the commands; from "tuck," to "go," which indicated we were out of the tuck position. Luckily, his impromptu strategy worked seamlessly as though we had practiced it that way all along.

But I was not ready to rejoice, because the most difficult part of the course was still ahead of us. A long, sweeping left turn was coming up. This was the section of the course where a skier could easily lose time, but thanks to Cliff's unexpected tuck command trick, it didn't happen.

The day before the snow conditions had been dangerously icy. Skis create a lot of noise on ice, making it difficult for blind skiers to hear commands from the guide and to detect other sounds that help us to gauge speed. Luckily it had snowed a few inches overnight, improving the conditions immensely. However, it hadn't snowed enough to erase the possibility of suddenly hitting a patch of ice, completely disrupting and disorienting a blind skier's balance.

In fact, as Cliff and I approached the steepest and most challenging part of the course, where two fairly tight turns were waiting for us, he hit a patch of ice just seconds before he was planning to call a hard right turn. Instead, he had to call, "check speed!" Unfortunately, there was not enough distance between us for me to slow down and avoid running into him. Luckily, we were so perfectly synchronized, all he had to do was widen his skis gently, so that my skis ended up right between his without causing a problem at all.

As we had practiced many times, when he saw me approaching, he gave me the command, "push off!" I pushed off of his back with my fists, with just the perfect amount of pressure to create enough space between us to maneuver the upcoming right turn. Executing that maneuver perfectly was the deciding factor in completing this race successfully. If the tips of my skis had not ended up exactly between the tails of Cliff's skis as they did, or if I had pushed off his back a little less or a little more, the outcome would have been totally different.

After finishing that section without incident, we were out of the danger zone and completed the remainder of the course in a tucked position, carrying as much speed as possible in the flat area all the way through the finishing gate.

Past the finish line, Cliff called, "hard left to a stop," kicked off his skis and ran over to give me a big hug. Nearly out of breath, he said, "We did it! We won! Nobody can beat our time now!" I could hardly breathe myself.

Now I found out why he had called the tuck command at the top of the course. In the four practice runs, we were always in the lead; however, in the last practice run, somebody came very close to our time. Cliff was not about to take any chances of finishing second. He decided not want to warn me ahead of time of his strategy, afraid that I would tense up unnecessarily and screw up. He also wanted to send a clear message to the other competitors coming down behind us that we couldn't be caught, so no sense in trying.

Two of my best friends, Anne and Agnes Gautier, had been watching the race from the middle of the course, standing next to the Swedish videographers. They immediately skied down to see me at the finish line. They pulled me into their arms and the three of us started screaming and jumping around in a circle like little schoolgirls. Quickly, a race official came over to yell at us, "There's a blind racer coming down the course! The entire hill must be completely quiet!"

Of course we knew that. We were just too exuberant and rudely had begun celebrating prematurely. We sat quietly on pins and needles, watching everybody in my category ski down the mountain. And as Cliff had predicted, we finished in first place.

CHAPTER 86

CLINT EASTWOOD STEALS THE SPOTLIGHT

After the official photographs and interviews at the bottom of the racecourse, we all left the slopes. Now Cliff and I needed to concentrate on the Giant Slalom that would take place in two days.

That evening, Cliff and I had dinner with my two best friends, Anne and Agnes, who were staying in an efficiency apartment with my sister-in-law, Michelina, the only family representative who was able to travel from New York to Sweden to watch me compete. Agnes had been one of my housemates in Monterey, California, for a couple of years when she and her brother, Gilles, were students of English as a Second Language at the Monterey Peninsula College. They had been my main transportation to the Kirkwood Ski Resort in California's Sierra Nevada mountain range in the early days when I was learning to ski. I was lucky enough to meet them and share a love of the sport, which strengthened our bonds as friends even more.

I was also extremely lucky to have Cliff May as my racing guide. Cliff was a fine-finish carpenter who lived with his wife, Chris, in Kirkwood, California, in a beautiful ski chalet he had built from scratch. He always kept his work schedule flexible so he could ski and train with me whenever I was available. Luckily his wife was always supportive of his passion and commitment, particularly when we had to travel to participate in races. He always paid his own travel expenses and never once asked me for reimbursement.

Cliff had become interested in guiding blind skiers through a special program sponsored by the Kirkwood Ski Resort. Their motto was: if blind people can find their way to the ski slopes, the resort would take care of the rest. This generous offer brought blind people into the sport who not even in their wildest dreams imagined it would be possible.

The excitement and exhilaration were contagious as blind people like me had the opportunity to enjoy the sport just like everyone else. Both blind and sighted people came out of the woodwork eager to participate in this activity. The blind ski program became a fixture at the resort for years to come.

I am one of several world-class skiers who are indebted to the Kirkwood Ski Resort for our success. In particular, I appreciated the work of Kirkwood locals, Ron Salviolo and Bob Webber, who contributed in a big way to the program for a number of years. To make the program successful and available to everyone, Kirkwood sponsored training for the guides, offered complimentary rental equipment, and provided lift tickets for skier, guide, and driver. Some of the local homeowners even threw in free lodging for everyone. It was nearly impossible not to fall in love with this exciting and glamorous sport.

That night after winning the downhill, while sipping a glass of champagne, we watched the local Swedish television coverage of the competition. It was shorter than we expected and not quite as thorough. Except for the Swedish athletes, hardly any of the other competitors received a mention. Immediately after that, though, the newscast began an extensive report on Clint Eastwood, who had just been elected mayor of Carmel, California.

"Hey, what about us?" Cliff interjected. "We just won a gold medal in the downhill and we're from California! I'll have to have a word with Clint about hogging all the news coverage."

I did take this lack of news coverage a little personally, but at the time the organizations for disabled athletes were only in their infancy. They had not yet earned the reputation required to get attention from international media. Perhaps at the time my feelings were hurt because I still had the need to prove something to the world. I was not yet comfortable with sticking my middle finger at my blindness as I am today.

CHAPTER 87

SAVORING A SPECIAL MOMENT

With one gold medal under our belt and the confidence that went along with it, on the 15th of April, Cliff and I won a second gold medal in the Giant Slalom. The Giant Slalom wasn't nearly as challenging as the Downhill race, but like every race it still rattled our nerves at the starting gate. We executed each turn perfectly. The snow conditions were excellent with no patches of ice or soft snow anywhere to be found. The course was shorter and without any particularly difficult sections. Cliff and I skied like champions and were confident about winning. By the time we crossed the finish line, Cliff and I were unbelievably grateful to have won both races with the fastest time throughout.

Once the race was over, Cliff looked at the scoreboard one more time to revel in our gold medal results.

"What the f___ is going on!" Cliff shouted.

"What? What?" I screamed in response.

"I can't believe this! It says that we have been disqualified!"

"Disqualified? What in the hell for? Did we miss any gates?"

"No," said Cliff, "we didn't make one single mistake. They better not be messing with us. Wait here. I need to get to the bottom of this immediately!"

"Don't worry, there must be a mistake," my friend Agnes said in an effort to make me feel better.

I felt sick. None of us could believe the horrible news on the scoreboard.

Cliff came back fuming. "They want us to wait while they investigate!"

"Our category is small. What is there to investigate? I don't remember hitting any gates the wrong way, or doing anything else wrong. Do you?"

Cliff took a while before he answered. "No, we did not make any mistakes at all. And if we did, it certainly was not obvious to me."

And so we waited, waited, waited, and waited some more; all the while reviewing the racecourse, trying to remember where we could have possibly made a disqualifying mistake. Neither of us could think of a thing.

Eventually, a race official approached us and said they had mixed up two bib numbers, and that the error belonged to another skier who wasn't even in our category. Cliff and I were, of course, relieved and were able to breathe as the adrenaline left us. And yet it wasn't quite over for me.

"Cliff, take me to the announcer's booth."

"Grab my arm; let's go."

We ran to the announcer's booth.

When we arrived, I said to anyone who would listen, "For the last hour my ski guide and I have been sick with anxiety, wondering what mistake we could have possibly made to be disqualified. You need to make a correction immediately, and make it loud and clear to the entire mountain!"

The announcer reassured me in his beautiful Swedish accent, "Don't worry, I will announce the correction." Moments later the entire mountain seemed to tremble at his very loud announcement correcting the error, asserting that indeed Cliff and I had finished in first place and won a second gold medal. He spoke it over and over, loudly and clearly, both in English and Swedish.

Late that afternoon we all attended the outdoor closing ceremony in full dress uniform: a blue wool blazer with insignia patch, white shirt, a gray skirt for women, and gray slacks for men. When my name was called, butterflies once again surged in my stomach as I walked onto the platform.

Now that the competition was over, I realized how unique and special this day was in my life. I was so proud to be winning another gold medal for the United States. While people applauded, I tried to savor every possible instant of this very special moment as I listened to the national anthem while snowflakes gently tickled my nose. I wanted to box up the entire experience and take it home with me. But I knew I could only take the uniform, the mementos, and the memories.

The closing ceremony ended with a banquet and the competition among international teams was replaced with a wonderful sense of camaraderie. It was heartwarming to see so many people with disabilities just relaxed and being themselves, without the competitive athlete personas they had embodied for the past weeks of competition.

A band played and we danced. A man with no arms asked me to dance. I remember being a little surprised when he said, "You have to grab my hook, and I'll lead you to the dance floor." Wow, I thought to myself, how impressive; this man knows how to invite and guide a blind woman to the dance floor.

Before the evening was over, in the euphoria of the moment, athletes who had been competing against each other for the past two weeks exchanged phone numbers and addresses, promising each other we would keep in touch. We all wanted the warmth and friendships to go on forever. Sadly, though, the next day we all had to pack up and head home, as this wonderful, one-of-a-kind experience came to an end.

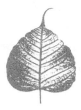

CHAPTER 88

SKIING FOR ITALY, 1988

"Wow, what an experience! It must have been tough going back to real life after that," Rosie said.

"You're right. It was extremely hard. I felt like I had fallen from a tall building into a deep crater," I said. "Those world championships were a hard act to follow. The only thing I had to look forward to was being reunited with friends and my German shepherd guide dog, McCloud, whom I had left behind for over a month."

"So what made you decide to switch to the Italian team; that's kind of curious," said Frank.

"After winning the gold medals, I thought I would be happy ending my racing career. I had been lucky enough to win, so I thought I should end on that high note and just enjoy recreational skiing. But as the 1988 Winter Olympics approached, my racing blood started to boil. The Olympics were going to be held in Innsbruck, Austria. I love Austria, and the more I thought about it an audacious idea crossed my mind. I am still an Italian citizen. I wonder if the Italian Federation for Blind Athletes would consider accepting me on their women's blind ski team? That's what I asked myself."

"Why didn't you stay on the American team? You were already on it," said Frank.

"I had already won for the Americans, and I thought it would be cool to try and win for my native country, too," I said. "There was only one way to find out if that was even possible. So I wrote an inquiry letter. Within a couple of weeks I received an answer saying that the Federation would be honored to have me on their team as well as my ski guide, Cliff May. I couldn't believe it! I was beyond ecstatic to be accepted, and luckily Cliff was more than eager for one more round of racing."

"Let's roast some more chestnuts so you can finish telling us the rest," said Frank.

"Go ahead, I always have room for more chestnuts," I said, as I continued my ski stories. In January 1988, Cliff and I flew to Italy for a few weeks of training with the Italian team before participating in the Olympics in Innsbruck. During the last few days I spent at work, my colleagues were filled with envy. "Lucky you, what a deal! To get an official excuse from work just so you can spend two-and-a-half months skiing in Italy and Austria."

"You're right. I am lucky. This time the Italian team is picking up my expenses, unlike the American team. But for me, by the time the whole thing is said and done, I will have gone almost three months without pay."

"Still," they would say, "just to get away from this place for three months is enormous."

I had been teaching Italian at the U.S. Army's Defense Language Institute in Monterey, California, since 1982, and except for a few rough patches here and there, I really enjoyed my job. Through my work I had been able to fully immerse myself in my beloved culture. In the Italian Department we never spoke English; and we gave military students an intensive language course so that in six months they would be ready to live and work in Italy.

For me, my job was the next best thing to be living in Italy again. I loved most of my colleagues and there were times when I even took them for granted, much like one does with family. The Defense Language Institute was also the place where I met my prince, a young French professor with a Ph.D. in 18th century French erotic literature. Neither one of us believed in Heaven or Hell, but serendipity brought us together to create our own terrestrial Heaven. With him, I was finally able to be myself without reservations. I discovered that unconditional love is not just something that poets write about and people dream about. I was actually lucky enough to find it.

My colleagues were right, I thought. The Defense Language Institute was not necessarily a teacher-friendly place, so the opportunity to get away from it for such a long stretch of time was phenomenal. For me, however, it was a bittersweet deal. I was feeling a tremendous amount of pressure within me to deliver a gold medal for the Italian team and I had no idea how to make that happen with certainty. The more I brooded about it, the less confident I felt. I really wanted to enjoy the sport and the entire experience of competing internationally again, but the obligations I felt made that almost impossible to do.

To say that the Italian Federation gave Cliff and me the royal treatment would be an understatement. Ferragamo designed and sponsored our dress uniforms (the same uniform as worn by the National Ski Team!); Trussardi designed and sponsored the sportswear and toiletries and also provided four pieces of luggage that we used throughout the entire stay. No fundraising was required of us. Every piece of equipment was provided by the same ski and ski boot companies that sponsored the Italian National Ski Team. Boy, did that feel good.

Ski lodges in Italy served gourmet meals at every sitting. I was impressed that I was never served a meal consisting of a simple sandwich or "food-on-the-go" during my entire stay. And we never skipped pear grappa after lunch, even if it meant hitting the slopes a little later.

The pressure was mounting. I had to win the gold for my native country, that's all there was to it. There was so much "buzz" around me because of my prior two gold medals that I could hardly handle it. People were impressed with my skiing and were confident I would win gold again. But could I? What if I didn't win? I almost regretted my decision to represent Italy. Every time I even thought about the possibility of losing, my feet would shiver in my boots. I would hit the slopes every day anticipating the agonizing feelings of guilt and loss if I should fail to win after all the pampering I was receiving.

Toward the end of January, Cliff and I joined the rest of the team on one of the buses that transported not only the athletes, but the entire entourage, including our food and kitchen staff, to Innsbruck, Austria, and our hotel in the Olympic Village.

There was such good chemistry among the blind division of the Italian team, it was hard to imagine we were there to compete, sometimes against each other. We bounced off of each other so well, it felt like being in the middle of a non-stop Seinfeld show. We were always eager to be done with tasks that kept us apart so we could return to this great camaraderie we had created. Cliff adapted so well and was so popular, I often forgot to translate for him. "It's so much fun watching you guys laughing and enjoying yourselves, that there's no need to translate," he would say.

Like in every competition, we went through the usual routine of getting to know the terrain and practicing gates, but when the first race approached, as always my stomach began to curdle. I was only too familiar with this awful feeling. I had hoped it would be easier or different the second time around. After all, I was a gold medalist. That alone should have given me enough confidence to surmount this sick feeling.

On the contrary, I had put myself in a position of such high expectations, it was having a destructive effect on my psyche. It seemed impossible to get in the right zone no matter what anybody did or said to me. I couldn't even rely on my zombie mode, that absent state of mind, to feel better. I simply felt awful.

The night before the first race, the assistant coach made a tactile map of the course. I looked at it with my hands and I tried to memorize the layout. Like I had always done in the past, I would break it down into three sections and memorize the number of gates as well as the position of each gate in each particular section. It seemed very useful, but not quite as good as an actual practice run. In the past, I always had a chance to practice on the actual racecourse at least once. This time, the Italian team officials decided to keep everybody off the snow the day before the race, thinking that it would be beneficial to our performance if we gave our muscles a rest. I disagreed, but I was overruled.

Before bedtime, the team doctor gave me some valerian extract drops to help me get a good night's sleep. Well, I didn't sleep at all. My mind was racing in every direction possible, but not on the racecourse. In the morning, I robotically did what I was supposed to do and hoped for the best. We received the usual words of encouragement as we moved toward the starting gate. Cliff reassured me that the course was a piece of cake compared to what we'd done in the past. He said the gates were far enough apart from each other and the snow was groomed to perfection so there was no reason to worry.

We bolted out of the starting gate in our usual style of cocky winners. At first, it felt good to be racing again. Going around the second turn, though, I felt the gate brush against my left leg. I thought maybe I had gotten a little too close to the gate. The rules for hitting gates with your skis state that as long as the tip of the ski stays on the outside of the gate, there's no penalty. But if it goes on the inside of the gate, you are to stop and go around the gate again. Otherwise, you are disqualified.

We did very well on the rest of the course. As we passed the finish line, spectators cheered loudly as the time posted on the scoreboard showed we were in first place. Cliff turned to me and said, "I'm really not sure how you hit that gate at the top. I didn't want to stop and lose time, but if your ski went on the inside of the gate, we're screwed."

Our first place standing on the scoreboard did not last long. It was soon replaced with DQ—disqualified. For the first time ever, Cliff and I had lost a race on a technicality. To make absolutely sure the gate keepers were right, the Italian officials filed a complaint and paid the hefty fee that went with it. But unfortunately, the gatekeepers were right.

We had lost and that's all there was to it. I felt sick and sad, even sicker than I had ever felt before. I just couldn't get over it. But for a moment I thought, "Why are you being so selfish? Let someone else bask in the glory, for crying out loud!" But that sentiment didn't last long. I'm not selfless like the Pope or Mother Teresa. I'm selfish and I wanted to win again, especially for my beloved native country.

"Why were you so hard on yourself?" Frank asked. "Nobody likes to lose, but you still did your best, so that's the way it goes. Sometimes you win and sometimes you lose."

"Yeah, he's right. Don't be so hard on yourself," added Rosie.

Sure! Easy for you to say. I could have tried to do my best all I wanted, but if I didn't win the gold medal, I would have been a big disappointment to everyone who had believed in me and supported me. Being a disappointment is a huge burden to carry, especially when you already have a lot of other burdens.

I said, "The worst part about losing was watching poor Cliff feel so guilty for not making the right decision in that split second, especially when we had to listen to the coach jokingly say, 'You guys had so much lead time, you could've stopped for lunch and still come in first.'"

It's easy for people to come up with possible alternative outcomes after the fact, but in this case, the only factor that might have changed things would have been at least one practice run the day before to engrave the pattern of the race course in my mind. That's how blind racers need to prepare instead of resting and stewing over the possibility of losing.

Nevertheless, my entourage still believed in me, supported me, and could not get enough of me. They had high hopes and their support felt good. Off the snow we laughed, we teased, we joked, we danced, we flirted, and we plotted on how to disable the competition. Laughter, laughter, laughter. That was the way the Italian team operated on and off the snow, a constant exchange of pleasantries and repartees. It was hard to imagine that within only a few days, this magical time would come to an end.

The second and final race was the Giant Slalom. We all tried to put the disappointment of the Super-G behind us and concentrated hard on the Giant Slalom. The expectations for a gold medal were now higher than ever. After all, in the last race we only lost because of a technicality, not because we didn't ski fast enough.

Cliff and I started the race with our usual optimism and butterflies in our stomachs. "This is it! Let's go for the gold!" we told each other. Everything was going smoothly until suddenly my left ski came off. This should not have happened. After all, we were not skiing at super-high speed.

Cliff quickly helped me put my ski back on, but we had lost precious time. It was difficult to continue and perform at the top of our game. I trembled and felt weak, discouraged, and sick. I knew right then and there that for sure we had lost the gold medal. We finished third, which gave us an Olympic bronze medal, but once again the gold eluded us.

And now, to feel better, we needed to find someone to blame. Perhaps the technician assumed that Cliff being so meticulous, precise, and always well-prepared, would certainly take care of the skis, but in my opinion, the team technician is where the buck stops when it comes to the malfunction of the equipment.

The closing ceremony came with its customary excitement and melancholy for all of us. Unlike me, for most competitors it was their first and last opportunity to participate in an event so magnificent.

The day-long ride on the bus back to Italy with my teammates was a non-stop party with laughter and fun all the way. Once we made it back to the Italian Federation of Blind Athletes offices in Modena and before we all disbanded, the president of the Italian Federation for Blind Sports graciously invited Cliff and me to remain on the team to compete in the next international competition in two years.

Cliff had already decided before the Innsbruck Olympics that he was going to retire from guiding. As for myself, I told the Federation president I would love to try one more time to win for Italy. But without a steady guide it was going to be nearly impossible to train properly before the competition. The president reassured me that the Federation would fly me to Italy two months early in order to train before the competition. They would provide me with a ski instructor/guide to train as much as I needed. Well, I thought, that seems very reasonable. In fact, it was an offer too hard to refuse, so I accepted."

"Well, we're all out of chestnuts, so I guess we will have to settle for a shot of cognac to hear the rest," said Frank. My mother was getting sleepy, so Rosie and I took her downstairs to her living quarters and helped her get to bed. We turned on the monitor and went back upstairs to join Frank and sip our cognac. Frank and Rosie didn't seem to be bored yet so I continued with my story.

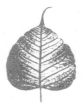

CHAPTER 89

"I AM DONE!"

In preparation for the World Championship in 1990, the Italian Federation of Blind Athletes had promised I would receive two and a half months of intensive training in Northern Italy at Federation expense. Unfortunately this training did not pan out as I had imagined.

The guide assigned to me was a ski instructor with fairly limited experience in working with blind skiers. Somehow the officials running the ski team were not well informed. They put far too much emphasis on the ski instructing and not enough on guiding techniques. He was authorized and paid to ski with me only two hours per day, which was a far cry from training with my previous guide, Cliff May. When Cliff and I trained together, we skied and worked on the slopes all day. This gave us plenty of time to practice various guiding techniques that would work best for us in competition. There were no long, leisurely lunches, and no waiting for fair weather.

Unfortunately this time around, except for the official days of training with the team, I did a lot of sitting and waiting, which was not a good thing for the psyche of an eager competitor who needed and badly wanted to win.

Two weeks before we left Italy to participate in the World Championship in Winter Park, Colorado, the Federation officials called an emergency meeting. At the meeting, the president announced as they were fine-tuning travel plans, they had realized there were too many people traveling for the funds available, so adjustments were in order.

You could hear a pin drop in the room. I'm sure people were squirming in their chairs, wondering who was going to be eliminated. After a long silence, the president suggested bringing along fewer guides to reduce costs. "Perhaps the B-1 skiers can share guides with the B-2 and B-3 skiers."

I nearly flew off my chair before he even finished speaking. I couldn't believe what he had just said. How could he come up with such a preposterous idea?

I said, "Excuse me sir, but before we go any further, I'd like to make one thing clear: I don't think the B-1s should share their ski guides with skiers from other categories. If anything, the B-2s and B-3s can share guides, because they have some vision. The B-1skiers do not! In the situation we are going to be facing, the B-1 skiers are going to need even more assistance than usual. The B-1 category consists of totally blind skiers who have no functional vision whatsoever. They are going to be traveling to a country where they don't speak the language. Furthermore, they will be in totally unfamiliar surroundings and under tremendous pressure to compete and win."

After my unexpected outburst, he was very apologetic and admitted his mistake. At that moment I realized that underneath all the fancy fluff, the lack of acknowledgement and respect for totally blind skiers existed in the Federation just like it did elsewhere. We were not often consulted or included in conversations that resulted in important decisions that affected us. This behavior has always infuriated me.

After the meeting, the team members came up to me and said, "Wow, what a performance! We didn't know you had it in you. Of course, you are in a better position to do that than we are. You don't risk losing much if they kick you off the team. After all, you've already competed in the past and won gold medals. Plus, you don't live here so they can't retaliate against you."

I responded that in my experience this situation was nothing new. Too many times decisions that directly affect blind people are made by those who know nothing about what works or doesn't work for us. If we want things to change, though, we have to speak out and fight hard, even when we have a lot to lose.

One morning in early March of 1990, the ski team was on the bus at the Federation for Blind Sports building in Modena, Italy. We were bound for the airport. The bus driver diligently loaded all the luggage and stacked all the ski equipment in the back of the bus. He climbed into the driver's seat and started searching for his keys. He couldn't find them. He traced his steps back and forth a few times. He opened and closed the back of the van time and time again. He looked around his seat over and over, but no keys. Then he asked, almost frantically, "Did anyone take my keys? This isn't funny. We are running out of time!" We reassured him that we were not guilty of such a crime.

A ski guide jumped out of the bus to help the driver find his keys. Still no luck. Then the driver looked at his watch and realized if he did not drive off right then and there, we would all miss the plane. Incredibly frustrated and nearly delirious, a barrage of colorful swear words directed at every saint, mother of Christ, and all of the dead popes erupted from his mouth. He sounded so colorful and poetic, I wished I'd had a tape recorder with me to memorialize it. I'm sure that it made every dead pope turn over in his grave and implore God to have mercy and help that poor driver of a van full of blind skiers find his keys.

A blind teammate then jumped out of the bus, asked the driver to open the back of the bus and methodically started feeling between all the layers of skis and bags. As he swept the bus floor, the top of his hand hit one of the keys sticking through between two skis. He separated the skis a little with his hand and the rest of the keys fell through. The driver had loaded the equipment on the bus without wearing his jacket. The keys had slipped out of his left shirt pocket and gotten trapped between the skis.

Nearly in tears, the driver grabbed the keys, jumped into the bus, and we took off. We didn't want to make light of the situation so we tried to stay quiet, but we could hardly wait to be together again where we could really, really laugh about the key incident and poke fun at the driver for not being able to find them.

Once on the plane, we discovered our seats were scattered amidst the other passengers. All of us were dressed in the official uniform of the Italian Federation and attracted a lot of attention from the other passengers as the flight attendants tried to distribute us around the plane to our designated seats.

Being separated was not acceptable. We wanted to sit together. We had lots of laughing to do. "Why? Why are we not seated together?" everybody kept asking.

No one seemed able to give us an answer until a flight attendant came up to us and said, "The reason you are scattered is that we cannot have too many blind people sitting together in case of an emergency."

"In case of an emergency? Are you serious?" some of us replied.

One of the totally blind skiers, armed with a wicked sense of humor and a degree in jurisprudence, became our spokesperson. "In case of an emergency?" he asked. "What do you think is going to happen to a group of blind people in case there is an emergency? We're not going to die any sooner than anyone else on this plane."

"No, no, no, it's not that, the problem is providing individual assistance in case there is a problem," the flight attendant explained.

"Listen to me," said the skier, "our life is a plane crash every single day. In case of an emergency, you will be glad that a bunch of blind people are on board, because we can provide assistance for you."

They finally gave in and we all got to sit together as one group. For the most part, the flight was another non-stop Seinfeld episode, providing lots of entertainment for those passengers who could understand Italian. In spite of the two meals they served on board, when dinnertime in Italy approached, stomachs started rumbling. The ongoing jokes and funny remarks were now heavily laced with moans of hunger. My teammates started referring to proper table settings and a typical mountainous menu with lasagna, or delicious polenta with wild mushroom stew, or venison. They were dreaming of meals they could eat when we arrived in Chicago.

"You guys are delusional," I said, "Get ready for fast food, and fast food only from this day forward, until the end of the World Championships do us part."

I then reached into my carry-on and pulled out some power bars that I always travel with because I know how unfriendly I can become to the world when I get hungry. Most of my teammates had never eaten a power bar, but they were hungry enough to accept them. They carefully scrutinized every crumb to make sure I wasn't feeding them horse manure covered in chocolate.

It was interesting for me to be part of a group of Italians who were extremely enthusiastic about visiting the United States for the first time. I tried to prepare them as best I could with useful information so they could feel at ease and enjoy their stay. This was the flip side of what I did for a living. Usually I prepared my students at the Defense Language Institute to live in Italy, but this time it was the other way around.

My useful information did not go far enough, though. Once we finally arrived in Winter Park, we spent quite a bit of time in a hotel lobby waiting for instructions as to where we were supposed to go next. One of the ski guides spotted a vending machine. I gave him some American money to use in the machine and away he went to get his drink. Seconds later, I heard him running outside, gagging.

"What happened?" I asked with concern when he returned.

"Smell this," he said, handing me a canned beverage. "Does it smell like beer to you?"

"Oh my god, no, this isn't beer. This is an American beverage called Root Beer. No wonder you are gagging. It's a soft drink. They would never sell regular beer in a vending machine in the U.S. You have to be 21 years old to consume alcohol here."

"Oh f___!" he replied, "what a drag!" and ran off somewhere to pour out the drink.

We spent our first day settling in and reviewing the schedule for the following two weeks. Once on the slopes, I was disappointed to see how unprepared the staff at the Winter Park resort was in hosting a large number of blind skiers and guides who did not speak English. The lift operators shouted and gestured as though that would bring about vision to the blind and English comprehension to all.

Unlike me, the members of the Italian team were very tolerant of ill-mannered people. But when it came to food it was a different story. After a few days of ingesting fast food or no food at all, everybody started becoming irritable and snappy. I tried immediately to patch things up by locating a supermarket and then a Chinese restaurant, for those who were more daring. That seemed to restore peace.

Here we go again, I thought to myself as we were queueing up for the Super Giant Slalom. It was a beautiful sunny day, no wind at all, a good day to win the gold medal; the only medal that seemed to have any significance in these competitions. My guide and I checked our equipment. I always wore my ski poles without the strap round my wrists, and for some reason I allowed my ski guide to convince me to do otherwise. "It's the rule; we don't want to be disqualified on a technicality," he said.

I wasn't sure about it really being a rule, but in any case it was a rule I never observed for good reason. If I fell, I wanted to be able to maneuver as quickly as possible without having to deal with ski poles attached to my wrists. Unfortunately I was overruled.

Well, wouldn't you know, half-way through the racecourse, I caught an edge and nearly fell. In trying to stabilize myself, I planted my right pole and the strap somehow pushed my glove half off. Before I could continue I had to stop, fix my glove, and grab hold of my pole. We completed the course but came in third. So much for the gold medal.

The Giant Slalom was scheduled for one week later. We practiced gates every day, but the practice course was short and did not resemble at all the course we would ski for the competition. We continued having fun on and off the snow, but frustration was mounting.

It snowed the day before the Giant Slalom, which suited us just fine. It's always great to ski on freshly groomed powder. As we were getting ready to practice one last run, my guide spotted the racecourse set for the next day.

"It's cordoned off," he said, "but do you want to take a chance anyway? We might get in trouble."

"I don't care about getting in trouble. If they want us to win, I need to try the racecourse at least once before the race. Isn't it obvious?" I said. "This is the only chance we have to review the racecourse."

"A skier from the U.S. team is doing it, so why not us?" said my guide.

"OK, let's go then," I said.

We left the run where the rest of the Italian team was skiing and headed toward the racecourse. We slipped under the rope, but as we drew closer to the starting gate, a race official chased us away. As soon as we returned to the team, we were reprimanded for not staying with the group. I tried to convince the coach it was crucial for B-1 skiers to be allowed to take at least one practice run on the actual racecourse before the competition, but to no avail.

Something snapped in me at that moment. This is a sham, I thought to myself. No wonder my category is underrepresented in these competitions. Totally blind skiers need to commit to memory the pattern of the race course in order to have the confidence necessary to ski their best. Right now, the day before the last race, they were denying us, the B-1 skiers, the opportunity to do the most essential thing that would help us win. Why hadn't our team officials arranged for at least one practice run on the actual race course?

This is a perfect example of occasional know-it-alls who make it to leadership positions even when they know very little about blind people and what works for us. This fight is never going to end for me. I can point things out to them until I'm blue in the face, but I'm never going to win this battle. I went to bed that night not thinking about the next day's race at all and I finally got a good night's sleep.

The next day as we were queuing up at the starting gate, my guide kept telling me, "Don't worry, we're going to do just fine. The course doesn't look that hard. We can win this."

Yeah, yeah, whatever you say. At this point we can win or lose. I don't give a shit. I no longer had the will or the confidence to win and I didn't care.

At the starting gate, my guide reviewed the direction of the first turn and reminded me, "Remember, I take off on the "One," and you follow me on the "Go." He proceeded with the usual last question before a race.

"Racer ready?"

"Ready."

"Three, two, one."

He skied out of the gate on the command "one," and I followed on the first command "go" as I had been doing for years.

Throughout the ski season I had noticed the radius of my right and left turns were not as consistent as they used to be. In December of 1988, I had suffered a fall which left me with some pinched nerves in my back. At times I experienced sudden pain, but I skied through it not knowing it was impacting my performance. I am not sure whether that played a role in this particular race, but it was certainly possible. Within a couple of turns at the top of the course, disaster struck. I hit a gate head-on with one of my skis, sending me into a forward somersault. Both my skis went flying over my head and past my guide.

My first reaction was one of relief. It felt so good to simply stretch out on the cool snow. The sound of silence was divine and peaceful. No more concentrating, no more ski commands to follow. But the best part of it all—to finally hear my heart and soul, along with every fiber of my body shout in unison, unequivocally, "I am done!"

I barely had time to take a full breath before a race official stooped next to me on my left side.

"Do you understand English?" she asked.

"Some," I replied, not moving a muscle.

"Are you hurt?"

"No."

"What country are you from?"

"Italy."

"Are you going to finish the race?"

"No," I said.

"Well, if you are not going to finish, then you need to clear off of the racecourse immediately, so the next racer can come down," she continued.

I lifted my head slightly, looked to my left where the official was squatting and said in my perfect California English, "Yes, ma'am, I know all that, but right now I just need you to get out of my face."

She stepped away, not saying a word. After a few moments, I turned onto my right side, tucked my feet under, planted my poles close to my right hip, and pushed up in one swooping motion, just like a pro. I walked over to the safety netting with my guide and together we slipped under to the other side.

"The bindings are cocked and your skis are to your right uphill. All you have to do is step into them," said my ski guide.

"No. I don't think so. I'm done skiing for the day," I said.

"What do you mean you are done skiing for the day?" he replied, bewildered. "We have to get down to the bottom of the mountain."

"You can ski if you want, but I'm walking."

Left without much of a choice and not heartless enough to abandon me there, he swung his and my skis over his left shoulder, grabbed my left pole with his right hand, and together, one step at a time, we walked down the mountain. There were a few firm hugs and soothing words from my teammates, but there were no "congratulatory" handshakes for losing, no thanks for trying, and no best wishes for the future from any of the officials.

And so, with a sour taste in my mouth, a sore body and a lump in my throat, I retired from ski competition.

CHAPTER 90

ROASTED CHESTNUTS AND COGNAC

I poured you another cognac," said Frank. "After hearing you describe that hike down the mountain, you need another shot."

"If I have another drink, I'll need assistance finding my bed."

"Don't worry, we won't leave you stranded sleeping in your chair," Frank reassured me.

"Wow, it must have been hard to retire like that," said Rosie.

"It was," I said. "I carried around a low-grade nausea for a long time, knowing that all of my efforts to make the sport and competitions for totally blind people better had gone straight into the toilet. But this happens from time to time throughout a lot of federations and organizations for the blind. Even in the workplace, blind people are often patronized, and they have to over-prove themselves to be recognized as valuable employees. Of course I'm not notorious for having patience, so I'm not always the best person to work toward necessary changes."

"You retired from competing, but that's when the fun skiing began for you, wasn't it?" asked Rosie.

"Yes; it wasn't long after that that Gilbert and I bought our ski condo at Kirkwood where you came to visit that one time," I replied.

"You were teaching a guide clinic while I was there," said Rosie. "It was fascinating to see you teach sighted skiers to lead blind skiers down the hill. You sure showed a lot of trust when you let the new guides practice by leading you down the slopes. Sometimes I was terrified. I didn't know if they knew what they were doing."

I said, "Initially they don't know what they are doing. What matters is that I know what I'm doing. I know how not to put myself in danger when I'm skiing with a new guide. By the way, there is nothing dangerous about skiing blind as long as the skier has good enough skills to respond to commands, the guide is properly trained, and they observe the safety guidelines. When I teach a weekend clinic, I send a manual to each participant to read ahead of time. First, I play a video that shows them how it's done and lets them know what to expect throughout the two-day clinic. Then the off-the-snow training begins. They take turns wearing a blindfold and being guided by an experienced guide through a maze similar to one that would lead up to loading the chairlift. We simulate loading and unloading of a chairlift, review all the safety guidelines, and practice the commands. In the final step of the indoor training they take turns guiding me through the maze. The next morning we repeat the process on the snow, including being guided down the hill while blindfolded. The final step is for each new guide to guide me down the slope. We keep repeating the process as we tackle more difficult terrain. We always have a debriefing at the end of each day to make sure all questions and concerns are addressed."

"Do you teach clinics anywhere in addition to Kirkwood?" asked Rosie.

"Actually, yes. Sometimes we teach at other resorts, including in Europe. We've done some in the French Alps and in the Dolomites in Italy."

"Getting back to your competitions; what's the top speed that blind skiers reach when they race? Do you know?" asked Rosie.

A lot of inaccurate information was floating around about that topic, so I took time to share my knowledge about it with my niece and nephew. First, in order to compete in blind racing, all the racers must be legally blind. But that doesn't mean they are all totally blind like I am. Those who fall into the B-2 and B-3 categories have some functional vision. The B-3s, in fact, have a lot of functional vision; enough to see the guide and several gates ahead of them. When you can see the guide and at least one gate ahead of you, you can anticipate the next turn more accurately. Therefore achieve a much higher speed than someone who is totally blind.

Only five percent of the blind population is completely blind. Unfortunately the public doesn't know those details. Some blind skiers with functional vision take advantage of this lack of knowledge to make their accomplishments seem more impressive than they really are. People in general love to create sensationalism or have people drool all over their accomplishments, so they are more than eager to brag about kicking ass down the mountain at seventy miles an hour.

But don't believe it for a minute, because for those of us who are truly totally blind, skiing above 35 to 40 miles an hour is unsafe. The noise from the skis and the wind make it impossible to discern accurate ski commands or other crucial information to ski safely. As for racing, the best strategy, particularly for totally blind skiers, is not to go as fast as you can and risk hitting or missing a gate and getting disqualified. Rather, totally blind racers should stay synchronized with their guide as much as possible, much like musicians when playing with an orchestra. The more synchronized you are, the better you perform.

"Well, I think the cognac is taking its toll on my consciousness. It's been more than a lovely evening. It's great to spend time with the two of you," I said.

"I'm getting tired, too. Thanks for all the great stories. We'll do it again tomorrow night," said Frank.

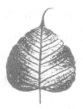

CHAPTER 91

GUIDE DOGS FOR MY MOTHER

The next morning, walking into the kitchen to have breakfast with my mother, I witnessed a scene more shocking to me than if Jesus Christ Himself had parachuted down to Earth and announced his candidacy for President of the United States. My mother was sitting in her chair petting, sweet-talking, and cuddling my magnificent German shepherd guide dog, Heinz! It was shocking only because my mother had always been vehemently opposed to having animals in the house. In fact, she had been opposed to the idea of my getting a guide dog in the first place.

How could the loving parent of a blind person oppose the idea of her child adding something to her life that would give her more independence, self-confidence, safety, and further happiness? Well, my mother had buried herself under layers of guilt and anger for having given birth to three blind children — for having, as she saw it, inflicted so much pain on them. Any reminder of our blindness was torture for her.

Whenever I was in public, the guide dog would naturally attract attention to my affliction, therefore heaping more shame and blame on my mother, something she would rather avoid at all costs.

"Why would you walk around with a dog?" she asked me years ago when I first informed her of my decision to acquire a guide dog. "People are not going to like it because not everybody likes dogs. You're going to be covered in dog hair and that would really make you look pathetic."

Hurtful comments like these, compounded by criticism, resulted in years of emotional distance between my parents and me. I could not penetrate their layers of guilt and overlapping ignorance no matter what I did or said.

For a long time I was convinced we would all go to our graves holding onto our self-righteousness. But here we were in 1999, with my mother directly in the path of one of the most feared and destructive diseases on the planet — a disease that wipes away your mind, leaving behind your body to waste away for years and years before you finally die.

And here she was, enjoying my dog. Had the disease already wiped away enough of my mother's mind that she was no longer inhibited? Was this her true self, the Rosa she was before piling on a ton of toxic guilt and regret? As she petted my dog's soft snout in her lap, she said, "He comes to check on me every morning to make sure I'm OK. He's so nice. He's better than a human."

I agreed. But I wondered how long the disease would allow me to enjoy my mother at this stage before it ravaged more of her mind. Was this the same mother who used to cringe every time she spotted a single dog hair on my clothing or on the carpet? Was this the same mother who once triggered one of the most violent emotional outbursts of my life?

On the morning of July 6, 1982, I called my mother in tears just hours after the death of my first guide dog, Colton.

"Ma," I said, sobbing, "Colton died!"

"What?" she replied, sounding shocked and worried.

"Colton died," I repeated, sobbing some more.

"Who died?" she repeated, expecting to hear the name of a human.

"Colton. My dog, Colton."

"Your dog Colton?" she asked.

"Yes!" I screamed, "He died early this morning."

"OK, OK, OK, calm down. Do you have to be this upset? I can't even understand what you are saying. Calm down. So, your dog died. You can get another one, can't you?"

I was in total shock to hear her say something so insensitive, but I wasn't surprised. I knew that I wasn't going to get an emotionally supportive response from her, but I just couldn't believe she was being so callous.

"Oh my God, are you going to cry this hard when I die?" she said, somewhat sarcastically.

That comment was just too much for me to bear. I slammed the phone down on her. I grabbed a hammer that happened to be within reach and smashed the hell out of my tile counter in total fury, pain, and disappointment. Lucky for both of us we were three thousand miles apart. The badly chipped counter remained in memoriam until the kitchen was remodeled years later.

Now that my mother seemed to be finally enamored with my dog, I decided to amuse her with some dog stories I had not been able to share with her before due to geographical distance and her lack of interest. I told her about that one time I went clothes shopping with an Italian girlfriend back in California. We decided to go for a quick lunch at a Chinese place because the service was fast and our time was limited. As soon as we were served, we asked the waitress to bring us the check along with a to-go box. We ate in a hurry, chatting at full speed. As soon as we finished the last gulp of food, we left the money on the table and bolted out of the restaurant walking arm in arm, as Italian women often do.

We were not more than twenty feet away from the door when we heard the waitress running after us shouting, "Ma'am! Ma'am! Ma'am, excuse me, ma'am, you forgot your dog!"

Heinz was an obedient dog who would stay put until I called his name and gave him a command. Furthermore, it was not unusual for my friend and me to go shopping without Heinz. Overwhelmed by haste, and distracted by our lively conversation, I had done the unthinkable. Yes, we had to face a full house of restaurant customers staring at us, wondering how in the world I could forget my guide dog. Well, I had.

My mother laughed and laughed over the story. "Was he waiting for you under the table?"

"Actually, he was standing when I walked back in, but he had not moved away from the table."

It was so new and pleasant to share a meaningful part of my life with my mother that I went on to tell her another dog story. During his university years as a percussion major at the Crane School of Music at the University of Potsdam, my brother Peter played the drums in a rock band most weekends. At that time he had his first guide dog, a German shepherd named Houdini, who was always with him when he played with the band.

One such time, when Peter was playing a solo during one of the songs, he heard the audience laughing, but he had no idea why. As soon as they finished playing, one of the musicians informed him that his dog Houdini had stood up, nonchalantly walked over to the stool where Peter kept his glass of beer, and lapped it up to the very last drop. Having quenched his thirst, he returned to his corner, lay down, happy and content.

My mother was hysterical, laughing, "Dogs drink beer? They don't find it too bitter? It doesn't taste like water." I was happy to see her laughing like that at a dog story.

While I was at it, since we were having so much fun, I decided to share another dog story. This one for sure, if I had told her just a few years earlier, it would have triggered a letter from her to the Pope asking him to excommunicate me. It happened in August of 1978, in Siena, Italy. I was on a trip through Europe with my good friend Connie, whom I had met during my junior year abroad in Avignon, France. The city of Siena was in full gear preparing for the Summer *Palio*, a traditional horserace.

We decided to visit the cathedral before the city became too hectic. As we approached the main entrance, a church official, whose job was to collect money and verify that the ladies' arms and shoulders were properly covered, started shouting at me, "You cannot come in! You have to leave the dog outside!"

"No," I responded, "this is a guide dog and by law he's allowed to go with me wherever I go."

"No, I don't care what kind of dog it is, it can't come in. It's forbidden!"

His response began to alter my blood pressure.

"Is he having a problem with the dog?" asked my friend, Connie.

"Yes, he is having a problem with the dog and I am having a problem with him," I responded. "When I tell you go, go. We are going to push our way in," I continued.

As we drew closer to the man, he began shouting louder. "This is God's house and animals are not allowed in God's house," he shouted.

Infuriated out of my mind, I shouted even louder, "Well, if animals are not allowed in God's house, then what are you doing here?" I pushed my way through, pulling Connie and my dog with me. The three of us took off running through the gargantuan cathedral — like racehorses.

"I'll have you arrested!" the man repeated over and over, trying to catch up with us. But then he had to turn back because he realized a lot of people were flowing through the entrance wearing shorts and halter tops and not paying. He had to decide which was the lesser of two evils.

Ironically, my mother was very amused by this story now, but if she had been there to witness it, she would have been so embarrassed and horrified at my behavior she would have disowned me.

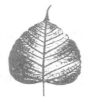

CHAPTER 92

NAVIGATING BLIND SPOTS

The next day, again during our usual morning coffee with my mother, we started talking about the past and about my brother Nic and his adventures. The first thing that came to her mind was his 40-day hunger strike and the toll it had taken on her.

"I couldn't believe he would do that. There were times in our lives when we didn't have enough food to feed our family and there he was years later, refusing to eat for 40 days for some cause that I didn't really understand," she said. "He could have died and devastated our lives forever."

I decided to redirect the conversation to a lighthearted experience that she had not heard about before. One year Nic came to California to spend Christmas with me and my husband. After the holiday shopping rush had calmed down, we all went to a men's clothing store to search for a particular item Nic needed. "I am looking for a warm shirt," he said. "In Brussels, everything is very expensive and I can never find what I want. I'm looking for something that would keep me warm indoors, but not quite a jacket. Maybe a quilted shirt or something like that." Once in the shop, my husband parked Nic and me by a rack of heavy shirts for us to look through while he scanned around the rest of the store to search for more items to choose from. It didn't take Nic long to come across a quilted shirt. "Bingo! I found exactly what I am looking for," he exclaimed joyfully.

Nic proceeded to remove his jacket, laid it on the rack and slipped on the newly found shirt. "This is perfect," he said triumphantly. "Unfortunately, it's way too big."

I walked over to him to feel the shirt, so that I could help him find more of the same one on the rack. In the meantime, my husband returned to our area and said, "I haven't seen anything that looks like what you are looking for. Oh! but where did you find the one you're wearing?"

"Right on top of this rack," Nic said. My husband joined us in searching for the same or similar shirt in a smaller size but to no avail.

Within a few seconds, a tall, large framed gentleman with a deep voice tapped Nic on the shoulder and said, "Excuse me sir, but you're wearing my shirt. Can I please have it back?"

It turned out the gentleman had left his own garment on the rack while he was trying on other shirts. "Oh, I'm so sorry!" Nic apologized profusely, while we all burst out laughing uncontrollably.

My mother was very amused and laughed heartily. "What a great repertoire of funny stories you have," she said. While she was still laughing, I decided to go for one that she was somewhat familiar with, but a bit more daring. I was not sure how she would relive it, but I took my chances.

In December of 1970, my youngest brother Peter was the only one still attending the residential School for the Blind in the Bronx, while Nic and I were both attending college. He was at Michigan State University, and I was at Harriman College in upstate New York. We were all three due home for the Christmas break at different times. Peter, now a senior in high school, was home first. Nic and I were supposed to be home around the same time. Once I got home, I inquired about Nic.

"Initially he was supposed to take the Greyhound bus, but then he changed his mind and told me that he would be driving home with friends. Hopefully that crazy guy will be home before Christmas," Mother said with some sarcasm in her voice.

Clearly she was not happy about that. She was worried about his safety riding in an old car in bad weather with a bunch of college kids.

The three of us looked forward to seeing each other now that we were no longer attending the same school or even living in the same town. We never spent money on long distance phone calls. We got news about each other only when we called our parents "collect" requesting money. Each time we got together now, we enjoyed comparing stories about the most outlandish experiences we had lived through since our last visit. Later that day, while chatting with Peter in our tiny music room, he shared a secret: "Did you know that Nic is hitchhiking home?"

"He's hitchhiking home? From Michigan? How do you know that?"

"He told me when I answered the phone yesterday, but he told me not to say anything to anybody."

I was both impressed and somewhat worried for him, but soon recovered. How dangerous could it be? After all, my friends and I certainly indulged in the habit. As much as we thought it was cool to be daring, as it got closer and closer to Christmas Eve, Peter and I started suffering from acid indigestion. Nic was simply not showing up.

"How long do you think it's going to take for him to get here?" Peter asked.

"I have no idea. It just depends on the type of rides he gets," I said.

Every time my mother would return from an errand, or just from stepping outside in the staircase for a short chat with the neighbor, she would ask us if Nic had called. We would reassure her that everything surely was fine. During the holiday season the roads were full of traffic and Nic and his friends were undoubtedly stuck in it.

"Don't worry. No news is good news," one of us would say. Even though our mother was worried sick, Peter and I decided we would not divulge the secret.

Luckily baking, cooking up a storm of everybody's favorite delights, and frequent visits from relatives and neighbors kept our mother distracted and occupied sufficiently that she avoided tumbling into total despair. Every now and then we could hear her voice coming from the kitchen imploring Baby Jesus for the grace of bringing Nic home safely.

While she fretted, my father would push back his chair, light a cigarette and walk outside to the street just to let off some frustration.

Perhaps he thought that going outside might bring Nic home more quickly. At least he felt that he was doing something. When he came back inside he would say, "He has no idea what torture this is for us. I hope someday his kids will do the same to him and we'll see how he will like it."

Christmas Eve was upon us in a flash, but still no Nic. The combination of worry, anger, and anxiety did not blend well with a festive dinner. "Why is he doing this to me?" my mother would constantly repeat as we ate. "I sent him money for the bus. Why is he making us sick with worry? I swear to God that I am never going to give him another dime in cash. Next time I will buy him the bus ticket myself. He should at least give us a phone call to tell us that he's safe."

"I'm sure he wants to call but it would take more time to look for a phone booth. And what if he doesn't have the right change? It's not like he planned to be late," I told her.

She would rant on and on, alternating threats with worries. She would get up from the table, walk to the stove to fetch the next course and constantly repeat under her breath, "Mother of God, please let him get home safely."

When it was time to go to bed, I couldn't believe we were going to sleep without Nic in the house. My mother had wanted to call the police, but Peter and I talked her out of it. However, we all agreed we would call the police if he didn't get home by 6:00 a.m..

At 4:00 in the morning, I woke up and decided to go check whether Nic had made it home. I was sure my mother had done the same all throughout the night. I was skeptical because I had not heard him come home, and it was not easy to get into our house quietly. I put my hand down on his bed and much to my surprise I found an ice-cold arm, immediately followed by a loud snort from his nose. Well, needless to say, I was relieved this nightmare was finally over; and I was particularly overjoyed that my mother could now relax and return to life as usual again.

Before 6:00 a.m., I heard my mother go to his room to check. After she realized he was all in one piece, she grabbed him by the foot and shouted, "Is this an acceptable hour to get home for Christmas? What kind of friends do you have who don't even care enough about their family to be home by Christmas Eve? Get out of bed, now! Go take a shower! Comb your disgusting long hair! Get dressed properly! You need to go to church and ask for forgiveness. If you don't you will go to Hell, you hear?"

After my mother had finished, my father came into Nic's room. "Nic, the telephone was invented for a reason! You had no excuse for making us sick like that. You poisoned our Christmas."

When the three of us were finally alone after Christmas dinner, Nic told Peter and me what had happened. "I started a couple of days ago in the morning thinking that with one or two rides I would make it to New York in one day. Unfortunately I forgot my cane in the first car, and I was only a couple of hundred miles into the trip. I thought the driver was going to realize immediately that I was without a cane, because it was right next to him on the seat, and that he would make a U-turn and bring it to me. Only he didn't.

"So, I looked around for a stick or branch to improvise, and did find something but you know, it's nearly impossible to get picked up when you are holding an improvised stick instead of a white cane in your hand. Especially when you don't make eye contact. They probably thought I was tripping on acid or something. I finally got a ride for a few more miles but it was almost dark. The guy who picked me up was nice enough to invite me to spend the night at his house so that I wouldn't freeze to death on the road. Before he dropped me off on the highway the next day, he helped me file down the branch so that it looked more like a beat up white cane.

"The last guy who picked me up gave me a ride all the way to the city. I then took the train to 241st Street where I was hoping to get a bus to Getty Square right away. Unfortunately, it was way after midnight, so

I had to wait a long, long time. I was afraid that I was going to have to spend the night on a bench on 241st Street. When the bus finally came I was the only passenger on it. I got off at Getty Square and walked home just in time to go to the six o'clock Mass, Ha Ha Ha."

Once the holidays were over Nic was anxious to get back to his girlfriend. He reassured my mother with all his might that he was going to take the Greyhound bus back to Michigan.

"I don't know if I should believe you," said my mother.

"I swear. I have to take the bus because none of the students I know who drive are going back yet," he said with conviction.

He asked my mother to make him two big meatball sandwiches for the road. He stuffed them in his backpack and with a new folding cane in his hand, he walked out of the house reassuring my mother he was on his way to the station to catch a Greyhound bus. Instead, he made his way to the highway and stuck his thumb out to hitchhike back to MSU.

My blind siblings and I wanted to live rich lives full of adventures and new experiences, so it was only normal over the years that we would withhold some information from our parents in order to protect our freedom and their peace of mind. Now I was regretting giving my mother the full version of the story. It was painful to see her agonizing over the worst case scenario, even 30 years later.

I could only imagine what her reaction would have been if she were to learn that her youngest blind son was one of those infamous college students who ingeniously figured out a way to use tones from an electric keyboard to bypass the AT&T billing system. Long distance calls were very expensive at the time, so there was always a line of students outside their dorm room waiting to call their parents for free. It became a calling frenzy.

Eventually they were caught. Thankfully they were fined but not arrested, thus saving my parents a great deal of grief. And for sure, her life as she knew it would end if I shared one of the most frightening moments of my life when an old boyfriend threatened to throw me off a 12-story building if I didn't submit to his sexual demands. And definitely she didn't need to hear the full details of Nic's 40-day hunger strike when he nearly died in an attempt to force the Belgian government to draw up a Marshall Plan that would reduce death, hunger, malnutrition, and abject poverty in the world.

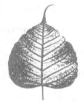

CHAPTER 93

HIJINKS ON THE HIGH SEAS

To change the mood I brought up a more light-hearted story that I knew she was partially familiar with, but we hadn't talked about for years. It was the story of my returning to the United States by ship in 1974, after studying abroad for a year. She enjoyed hearing about my various travels, but this particular trip had a special place in our hearts. Now that she could no longer scold me over some of the details, I felt safe reminiscing about it with her.

I had spent the academic year of 1973–1974 in Avignon, France. When the school year ended I enjoyed some extensive summer travel in Italy, ending my stay with our old landlord and family in Naples. As the return date to the United States approached, I wrote to my parents expressing the desire to travel home by ship rather than by plane, not only for the experience, but for the low student rate.

My parents had categorically rejected the idea, concerned that it would be unsafe for me to travel alone on a ship and proceeded to send me a non-refundable, one-way plane ticket. I immediately returned the plane ticket with a letter saying, "If you don't send me a ticket to return to the United States by ship then I just won't return home."

It was early August, and I still had a month to go before I had to be back in the States, so I had no trouble leaving my parents stewing over my letter. I knew that sooner or later they would come around. After all, I really didn't think they had it in them to leave me stranded in Italy. As I predicted, within a couple of weeks I received a one-way ticket to travel home by ship, as well as a letter filled with reprimands. My mother wrote, "You never change. You were born with the devil in you and you still have the devil in you, no matter how old you get. Even after a year away from us, you manage to bring us aggravation."

On August 29, 1974, I embarked from Naples on the *Raffaello*, scheduled to arrive in New York eight days later. When I boarded the ship the captain imposed one rule that applied only to me, not to the rest of the passengers. "*Signorina*, we are very happy to have you on board and we want to make sure your eight days with us will be a wonderful experience. However, I have one request: to make sure you are safe, a crew member has to know where you are at all times."

The crew was mostly composed of young Italian men, so I was actually flattered and had no trouble following the rule to have at least one crew member escorting me or checking on my whereabouts at all times.

I shared my stateroom for four with a South American nurse/nanny, Lia. She was about my age and was traveling with a countess who had a newborn. She and I became friends immediately. She ended up spending all of her time with me whenever she wasn't working for the countess.

Within the first day or so, an Italian-Canadian gentleman traveling with his family quickly befriended us and became almost a nuisance following us around, particularly in the evening when he would show up at the club without his wife and insist on dancing with us the entire evening.

One day after thinking long and hard on how to get away from him, Lia and I informed him we were turning in early for the evening. Instead, we went to our stateroom and fussed around with our various outfits for some time until we thought we were disguised well enough to fool the gentleman. When we got to the club Lia saw him sitting at the bar, so we selected a table as far away from the bar as possible. He nursed his beer for a while; then after less than an hour, much to our delight, he disappeared. At last we were able to mingle with some single men our age and have some real fun.

Earlier, before we entered the nightclub, I had a conversation with Lia about what often happens to blind women in nightclubs. "Generally speaking, Americans are much slower at interpreting body language than people in other countries. In the States, if I fail to make eye contact with people, or if they fail to see my cane or guide dog, they automatically assume I am drugged or spaced out rather than blind. But the most frustrating thing occurs in nightclubs. I love to dance and unless men see me on the dance floor, dancing up a storm, they won't ask me to dance because I don't respond to their visual invitation. I hate to have to prove myself all the time, but that is the reality.

"Tonight this will be our strategy. If you see someone approach whom you think is going to ask me to dance, start talking to me so that you can easily insert information such as, 'coming up on your right or your left,' so that I can turn towards him and accept his invitation if he asks. Once I hear where he is, I'll grab him and take care of the rest."

"Wow, I'm going to have fun doing this," Lia said. "I'll make sure you are on the dance floor before me. In case you happen to be dancing with a numbskull who forgets that you are blind and walks away from you at the end of the dance, I'll make sure you get back to the table safe and sound."

Lia and I finally had a chance to be on our own, have a good time and enjoy ourselves that evening. We danced a lot and even managed to meet some single guys. The next day, the overbearing Italian-Canadian man caught up with us and said, "You ladies missed out on a good night of dancing. We were up until two in the morning."

"Good for you," I replied. "Maybe this evening you can do that again."

When I went to dinner the next evening, I ran into a gentleman I had danced with the night before. He asked me if I would like to join him for a cocktail later on. I accepted and told him I would meet him at the bar when the music started. Lia was working that night so I notified the steward I would want someone to escort me to the bar later. Once I arrived at the bar, my date was already there waiting for me. After a few drinks and a lengthy conversation, he asked, "Would you like to go to the upper deck and observe the full moon?" I accepted.

We were the only passengers out on the deck. I welcomed this sublime experience of glorious sounds of the sea, uninterrupted by noisy and sometimes ill-mannered humans. We leaned on the railing in silence. It was great. After a few moments he drew closer to me, the side of his head nearly touching mine. "Can you see how big and bright the moon is?"

I paused briefly. "Yes, I can," I replied softly. "I can see the moon, but I can't see the stars."

We stared at the sky for a few moments without talking. He stepped back and whispered, "Come with me, I'll take you closer to the stars."

He took my hand and guided me to a set of narrow stairs. With each upward step, the world underneath my feet felt smaller and smaller. By the time we reached the crow's nest, the immensity of the sky and the ocean became my new world. I felt so small in the majesty of these surroundings. The ship under my feet was a microscopic speck of nothing. The bright full moon above caressed our faces with her soft silver light. I tried hard to imagine the immensity of the universe. The two of us looked as though we were posing for the most romantic picture ever. The only thing missing was a kiss and a few butterflies in my stomach. After a few moments the kiss came, but unfortunately, no butterflies.

When we'd had enough of posing for romance without any magic, we disassembled the love scene, carefully descended the narrow stairs and went back inside, bypassed the bar, and walked around the ship for a while. Since we were both traveling students without much money, we decided to save on the cost of drinks at the bar, and eventually ended up in his stateroom for a shot of cognac.

Within a quarter of an hour, we heard the hurried and heavy footsteps in the hallway of crew members asking around, "Has anyone seen the *signorina*?" I had unintentionally fallen off the radar. When my roommate, Lia, came back from her shift with the countess' newborn, she had innocently asked our steward if he had seen me, and that sparked a panic on the ship. The *signorina* was missing!

Soon the announcement came on the intercom: "Attention all passengers and crew: At the moment we are trying to locate the *signorina*. If anyone has seen her, please notify a member of the crew immediately." Now I was completely mortified. Something needed to be done immediately to put out the fire.

My gentleman friend reassured me, "I'll take care of it. Don't worry." He slipped out into the hallway quietly, approached one of the stewards and whispered in his ear, "I found the *signorina*. She is with me." Shortly after, the announcement from the captain came that the *signorina* had been found safe and sound.

During the first six days of the trip we had enjoyed calm seas and beautiful sunny weather. Two days or so before docking in New York, though, we learned we were approaching the outskirts of a hurricane. Little by little, the ship began rolling more and more vigorously. Crew members secured ropes everywhere so that the passengers would always have something to hold onto. *Finally! Some real excitement!*

Not everyone on board shared my sentiments and in fact, many passengers began to panic. The captain made reassuring announcements on a regular basis, but it provided little comfort for those who preferred popping valium and other sorts of tranquilizers to stay calm. The evening entertainment proceeded as usual, but no one dared to dance or move around if they could remain securely seated.

When the band played one of my favorite waltzes, I suddenly couldn't resist. I jumped up and shouted, "I need a courageous dance partner!" To my disappointment, the one who rose first was the Italian-Canadian man that my roommate and I had been trying to avoid for days. He did know how to waltz, though, so I was grateful. It didn't take us long to get into the perfect rhythm, lengthening and shortening our steps with the rolling of the ship. We kept a perfect tempo throughout the entire waltz, which earned us a loud and lengthy applause at the end.

At eight o'clock the morning of September 5, 1974, we docked in New York Harbor. A few hours later, dressed in the latest Italian fashion and escorted by a charming young steward, I disembarked the *Raffaello*. "Here she comes, Miss *Italia*!" I heard my mother exclaim from about ten feet away. She ran towards me and held me in her arms.

"You are so tan, you look fabulous. Did you have a good trip?"

"Everything was wonderful; I loved my time on the ship. See? Nothing happened to me and I'm still in one piece," I said as we hugged and kissed.

"Yes, I know; you are courageous and you always get your way," she said happily.

"What in the world did you bring with you?" she asked when she saw my luggage arrive, consisting of two big suitcases and three large cardboard boxes.

"Lots of goodies that the relatives in Basilicata sent you. The week before I got on the ship, I went to cousin Antonio's wedding, remember?"

"You actually managed to go to the wedding?" my mother said with envy, wishing that she could have been there.

As soon as we arrived home we unpacked the cardboard boxes. My parents were overjoyed to see what I had brought back. Finely ground polenta flour that my mother had been trying to find in the U.S. for years. Sheep's milk cheese, so reminiscent of our time on the farm. And cranberry beans that had been harvested just a few weeks earlier.

"This is the next best thing to being with our relatives in Basilicata," my father said with a big smile in his voice. "We have enough beans to share with all of our relatives here in New York, so we can keep the tradition alive by planting and harvesting them every year, just like we did back in Basilicata."

"I could have never brought all these treasures with me if I had returned to the United States by plane," I reminded them.

"I know, you are right, you are right," my mother said with tears of joy.

My mother really enjoyed revisiting this story with me. It had been 25 years since we had talked about this trip. She had no trouble remembering every detail about my cousin Antonio's wedding as I had described it 25 years prior. For every one of our relatives that I mentioned, she reminisced with accuracy about her past experiences with them, their lives, and family histories, including gossip.

She was immediately aware if I confused people's names and corrected me. She talked about the entire wedding with such relish that I wished for her sake that she could have been there instead of me. She showed no sign of Alzheimer's as we talked about the wedding. But at the same time she showed no recollection of my father's death just a week earlier. At least not until I mentioned bringing back the dried beans that my uncle Domenico (my father's brother) had sent with me.

"Isn't it nice that a lot of our relatives here are still planting and harvesting the beans I brought back in 1974," I said. Her mood slowly became more somber.

"You have no idea how many times your father told the story about the beans you brought back from our hometown in Italy. He shared them with anybody who was willing to plant them in the spring, harvest them, and enjoy them a few months later," she said with pride, her voice breaking at times with sadness. Her memory had been jolted into the present, and she remembered that her husband, my father, was no longer with us.

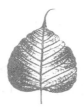

CHAPTER 94

COMING TO TERMS

When I flew to New York to attend my father's funeral on the twelfth of January, 1999, I had no idea I would end up spending well over a month with my mother.

For the most part, it was just the two of us. It gave us a chance to reminisce about the past and reset the tone between us, which had not always been pleasant. I had never spent that much time alone with my mother so it was precious, but also painful. I had never dreamed I would be physically present to witness the inconsistent behavior caused by Alzheimer's in my own mother.

At times her memory seemed sharp and normal, but at other times it would seem as though she had forgotten that she had blind children. Occasionally she would show me a photograph and expect me to see it. Sometimes she didn't even recognize herself in family pictures. My father had died suddenly and now I was slowly losing my mother.

As we finished our leisurely breakfast on one of the last mornings I spent with her, I heard her shifting in her chair. She put her left elbow on the table, resting the left side of her head in her palm facing me. I knew this pose. It always meant she was about to say something heartfelt. But this time it was even more than that.

"We could keep on talking forever and I would never learn all the crazy and wonderful things you kids did over the years," she said. "You learned to do so many things so well; more than I could have ever imagined. All my worry and anguish when you were little was so unnecessary. If only we had known then what we know now, life would have been so much easier for everybody. Ignorance is the worst affliction of all. You kids did well in school. You all learned to play musical instruments. You learned to speak many languages. You traveled to many parts of the world. All three of you became professionals, independent, and self-sufficient. And you, Carmela, even learned to ski, compete, and win medals. I couldn't have learned to do all those things, even if I had gone to school like you did." She finished with a solemn, even sad tone as if she were wishing she could do it all over.

"Ma, the day I stop traveling, the day I stop playing the piano, the day I stop teaching, or stop skiing, no one will ever notice the difference. But trust me, the day you stop making your homemade bread and homemade raviolis, the world will never be the same."

"Now, you're exaggerating. Do you really think so?" she chuckled with a big smile in her voice.

"Yes, I really think so," I answered. She remained in the same pose, gently tapping the fingers of her right hand on the plastic liner covering a hand-embroidered tablecloth. At that moment grief finally overtook me. With a heavy heart, hiding the tears in my eyes from my mother, I slowly walked away from the table toward the bathroom and turned on the light.

Through my big tears the light looked blurry and shapeless, bringing back one of the most painful memories of my life. I had been five years old when my parents took me to the residential School for the Blind for the first time. The reception room was illuminated by electric lights, something I had never seen before. I was amazed at how well I could see around me. The little bit of vision I had went a long way with electric lights, almost like being outside in the sunshine.

I kept staring at the wonderful light in the ceiling as my mother sat me on a big table in the middle of the room. I was surrounded by staff members who played with me and fussed over me. My parents were hoping that the many distractions and the attention of the staff would keep my focus away from them as they tip-toed out of the room. I quickly realized the truth. My parent were not going to stay with me at the school. My eyes filled with tears and the light in the ceiling suddenly became blurry and shapeless.

What a heavy price everyone in my family had paid for a physical disability that turned out to be little more than a nuisance. When we were young children, my parents, along with my two older sighted siblings, Benny and Maria, had devoted all of their energy towards mitigating what they had initially interpreted as a family tragedy. Nic, Peter, and I received an intense formal education that opened many doors for us. Benny and Maria did not have this opportunity. Although they became financially successful through hard work, they missed out on the carefree adventures of youth, the freedom to grow up at their own pace, the opportunity to explore their own talents, and to live life with the fervor my blind siblings and I enjoy.

This is my family's story. There had been difficult times. There would be more ahead.

I closed my eyes and wondered what my mother would be like when I returned to New York for my next visit. Would she still remember me? I had lived away from home since I was five years old and had said many painful goodbyes to my parents. Was this the last conscious goodbye I would share with my mother? I felt a heavy sense of regret for the many clashes and emotional outbursts over the years between my parents and me.

As for the future, watching my mother lose her memory and forget all of us would be difficult for my siblings and me. We would have to rely on one another for strength and support.

"You can speak your mind and say what you need to say to each other, good or bad," my mother had told us over and over whenever she caught us fighting or arguing. "But no matter what happens, never stop talking to each other because you are family. Remember that!" I had never given this advice much credence. It just sounded like something any mother would say, but now it was taking on a new and important meaning.

Having lived away from the family for so long, Peter, Nic, and I had had endless opportunities to embrace ideas that were foreign to those of our family. In fact, at times we felt like strangers at family gatherings. We had to change our behavior to fit in — almost as if immigrating again — as we straddled two worlds.

In the end, none of that matters. Our mother's simple wisdom would win out. We are a family, no matter how different we are from each other. We will get through this together. I wiped away my tears and went back into the kitchen.

"Ma, another coffee?"

"Yes, why not?" she replied.

I never had to convince my mother to have another cup of coffee. She loved it as much as I did, so we enjoyed another cup.

Later on in the evening before we turned in, my mother glanced out the window and said, "Wow, it looks like there is a full moon tonight."

"Is there?" I asked. "Do you want to step outside for a minute to look at it?"

"Are you kidding me," she replied, "It's freezing outside."

"There's no wind. It's not that cold. We will only be outside for a few seconds," I said.

I helped her bundle up and we stepped outside her kitchen door. Of course I couldn't see the moon any more like I did when I was a child, but I wasn't about to tell her that. I didn't want to disturb the peace of mind she had finally found as a result of Alzheimer's disease — beginning to forget that she had blind children.

The night air was crisp and still.

"Wow, it's a full moon all right," she exclaimed. "When we lived on the farm back in Italy, years and years ago, whenever we had a bright full moon like that during the summer, we used to work in the field at night to avoid the heat of the afternoon sun."

"Oh yeah, I remember that," I said.

"You do? How could you possibly remember that? You were so young at the time."

"Yes, I was young, but I still remember."

"Well, I wouldn't put it past you. You always seem so good at remembering everything," she chuckled.

Surprisingly she was not fussing about the chill in the air. This seemed to be a happy moment for her and I was glad. She looked up at the sky again.

"Wow! Look at the stars! There are millions and millions of them, and they go on and on forever. You can see them, can't you?" she asked.

I paused. I then looked up at the sky and said, "Of course, I can … I sure can …"

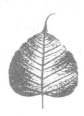

ABOUT THE AUTHOR

Blind since birth from Retinitis Pigmentosa, Carmela Cantisani is a native Italian who has made her home in the United States since she immigrated here with her family at the age of 13. She pursued a career in romance language teaching. She competed in one Winter Olympics and two World Championships for the disabled, winning three gold and two bronze medals in downhill skiing in the totally-blind category. Accomplished pianist, world traveler, and an excellent cook, Carmela developed and marketed her own line of gourmet salad dressings.

Carmela is the author of articles published in the Italian ski magazine *Sciare* and in *La Folla di New York*. She currently lives in Carmel, California, with her husband and her guide-dog.

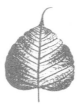